As I make the final edits on this book, the 2015 Reebok CrossFit Games is on television in the background. If, like me, you were an affiliate gym when the first Games was staged, you'll appreciate how miraculously our passion has spread in less than a decade. CrossFit has changed the way the world thinks about exercise. Not by watering down the definition of "fitness" to increase participation rates; nor by reclassifying "shopping" and "strolling" as exercise. No, the brand has changed the context of fitness by pushing the ragged edge of possibility.

JFK's famous speech on September 12, 1962 challenged the nation to put a man on the moon by the end of the decade. It was an outrageous challenge because it pushed the edge of possibility. But innovation requires outrageous challenges, not relaxation of standards. The "man on the moon" goal created the momentum to eventually launch the rocket. Rocket scientists had already been working to catch the Russians in technology, but refocusing on the audacious goal shot the nation's science to the forefront. As JFK said,

"We choose to go to the moon not because it's easy, but because it's hard."

No one knows this better than a box owner.

Before CrossFit, many "fitness professionals"--me included--

thought we'd solved the puzzle. But CrossFit wasn't just the missing piece: it was a whole new picture. This new definition of fitness is our "moon shot:" the inspiration required to change our universe. But there's a major difference: JFK already had rocket scientists. They required a deadline, and a big goal, but they already knew how to make things go "boom!"

For many affiliates, the inspiration came first. And that's fine; we're starting with "why" instead of "how." And a gym is very easy to start: an essay, a cool name, and a licensing fee smaller than a monthly car payment. We already know how to press the "launch" button.

The trouble is keeping the rocket in the air. Forget about landing on the moon: what happens when the rocket is ten feet up?

The world is watching our rising starship. Some are waiting--hoping, even--for a crash. The crash won't come from athletes: we continue to get faster, stronger, better. But these are the astronauts, not the scientists. We, the owners of thousands of small gyms, need to build ships that can reach the moon and, as JFK said,

"...deliver a man safely back to earth."

This means a sustainable business that will provide its owner with the money, sleep and joy necessary to inspire. It means a 30-year machine that can be turned over to your kids, so they can coach the children of your current members. It means the creation of wealth: a high value for the time spent. It doesn't mean short-term patches, like coupons or discounts, but the relentless pursuit of business excellence.

It means drawing a blueprint, then tightly turning every screw before lighting the match. Luckily, I've done the first part for you. This book, combined with Two-Brain Business and Help First, is the blueprint. Directions on turning the screws and the shared experience of other rocket scientists can be found at www.twobrainbusiness.com.

This book was written to educate and inspire. The educational pieces are driven by data, not dogma--you won't find untested "advice" here. The inspirational pieces are my own extensive (and very expensive) experiences as a gym owner. Most valuable of all are my mistakes: laugh at them, learn from them, and save the money and anguish I've already spent.

Work until you're happy. Then stop.

Chris

For my kids,
and for yours.

Table of Contents

Preface:

Two-Brain Business was published in 2012. Compiled from over 400 blog posts on DontBuyAds.com, 2BB started as a "greatest hits" handout at my first seminar. I was invited to share the speaker's podium with some (then) big names in the gym industry. One of the others had won the CrossFit Games; another had just opened his sixth franchise. I had nothing on these two, so I self-published Two-Brain Business and shipped 30 copies to the host gym.

That first batch had a hand-drawn head on its green cover. It was imperfectly edited, lacked a table of contents and the pictures didn't line up properly. But it was punk: the DIY nature made it somehow even more legit to the readers, as they'd tell me later. Like a homemade sample tape, Two-Brain Business was never supposed to be the "studio cut." But I got busy.

Within a few months, I started getting emails asking for help. As I sit down to write this update, my knowledge has been upgraded by conversations with over 800 gym owners. All one-on-one, and all on my dime. Over 10,000 hours' worth of testing, trials--and sometimes tears.

Two-Brain Business 2.0 isn't a sequel; it's an upgrade. It took me three years to record the audiobook version of Two-Brain Business, and I realized some of the information was outdated. Some was simply no longer true, and some had been refined by the hundreds of gym owners testing my theory in their real-life labs.

This is what I know to be true now. Each strategy and every tiny tactic have been proven to work in gyms around the world. 2BB2 contains less theory, fewer stories (though I've kept a few great ones) and more actionable items. And a table of contents, too.

Thanks for every email, every phone call. Thanks for lugging your book to my seminars, asking for an autograph, and being sincere when I look struck dumb. I think we're in this together.

Thrive,

Coop

What is Wealth?

It's not the yacht. It's not the gold watches, white beaches or private jets. Those might be the ways wealth is enjoyed, but they're not what makes you wealthy.

It's not self-fulfillment, either. Wealth can provide the time to seek your inner self, or free you from the basics (like fear and hunger) to pursue self-actualization. Wealth is means to an end for some, an end for others, and undefined for most.

Wealth can be simply stated as an equation: income / time.

The ratio of money earned to time required to earn money is the measure of wealth. The greater the ratio, the wealthier you are. This can mean a very high income, or a very low amount of time invested to create that income. It's not the total earned, but the value of each day, each hour, each minute spent earning. As your time increases in value, you become wealthier.

Wealth isn't freedom, but can create freedom. This might mean the freedom to work from home, or donate to a charity or watch your kid play baseball. Or it might mean a bigger house or other luxury. Those are the choices created by wealth.

There are many myths about wealth, of course.

Myth: wealthy people are greedy or evil. Truth: greedy people are greedy. Evil people are evil. Wealth simply provides more opportunity to pursue their greed; more leverage with which to ply their evil. But good people are still good, and wealth creates greater opportunity for their good.

Myth: people with kids are the wealthiest people of all. Truth: people who don't deprive their kids of time or money are the wealthiest of all. I have many friends with plenty of money, but no time. Many are business owners who work 70 hours every week and don't get to eat breakfast with their kids (this used to be me.) Conversely, I made friends in villages in Kenya who can spend all day with their kids, but can't guarantee a breakfast before school. Hollywood and Hallmark have romanticized wealth in two other ways related to emotion. Myth: Money doesn't buy happiness. Truth: It creates the opportunity to pursue happiness. I drive to work at 4am most days. I'm listening to country music, drinking coffee, and writing in my head. I like early mornings. I also like a nap after doing CrossFit with my friends in the noon group. My business dictates the 4am start, but wealth makes the workout and nap possible.

Myth: love is all you need. Truth: It's not all you need. You need to eat. I'm a strong believer in Maslow's Hierarchy of Needs, which explains the order in which problems must be solved. Love is even better on a full stomach. Take it from someone that's tried it both poor and wealthy: it's better with money.

Where does wealth come from?

If we agree that wealth is the value (measured by net income) divided by your time, then we can simplify the creation of wealth: spend less time working for the same money, or earn more money for your time. Simple--but not easy.

Knowing the equation doesn't solve the problem, but it does provide a way to find a solution.

Every week, I speak with 30 gym owners for an hour each. These are usually folks who are working hard: they're putting in long hours at the gym, helping people. Few got into the business to get rich (and most never will.) They're all gym owners because they wanted to help more people, or help the same people better.

Want proof? I've been on these calls with over 800 owners now. I've surveyed 2000 more. When asked, "What's your perfect day?" I've never had one say, "I wouldn't go to the gym." That's profound. Given all the time and money in the world, they'd STILL show up for their 8am appointment and teach someone to squat. Go ahead: try to name any other job in the world with that kind of love and commitment.

But most of these owners are focused on one side of the "wealth" equation: earning more, period. Maybe, like me, they have to pay the bills before they worry about luxuries like sleep. Or maybe they're trying to earn enough to pay a staff person so they can sleep in on Fridays. In a very few cases, they're simply goal-driven people who don't know what else to do.

Wealth doesn't mean a Rolex. It means the ability to buy a Rolex...or the ability to spend the day building a new playground at your kid's school. It means having $10,000 to spend on a watch...or to travel to Kenya and build a school there. I won't judge how you spend your wealth. My job is to create that choice for you.

Aren't Rich People Evil?

Most people are scared of money.

They don't understand it, so they don't talk about it. They don't have it, so they're suspicious of those who do. It's a cognitive bias: "That guy isn't smarter than me. He doesn't work harder than me. He must be cheating somehow."

When I write about wealth in this book, I'm writing about the value of your time. Your value is determined by how many people you help, and how much you help them. If you can change the lives of 10 people, what's that worth? How about 100 people?

If you can positively change the outlook, lifespan, health and love lives of a thousand people, do you deserve to be a millionaire? To work less, be as generous as you want and have a pool for your kids?

Is generosity ONLY good if it hurts you somehow? Will your clients be better served by a martyr than by a millionaire? Of course not. If you have all the money you need, you can give more value to your clients; more experiences to your kids; and more money to deserving charities.

Money is a tool. It's not "the root of evil"--evil is the root of evil--and it's nothing to fear. Do greedy and corrupt people have money? Sometimes, yes. But the best way to affect change in our world is to put the money into the hands of caring people making positive change. That's you, my friend.

"Once you make the distinction between money for independence and money for status, the rest becomes easy." – Nassim Nicholas Taleb

This book will guide you toward wealth. Not ostentatious wealth; not greed; not unfair practices. I'll talk about what's possible because comparison is our nature, and if you're only comparing yourself to the unwealthy, you're winning too easily. You're placing the bar too low. How much training do you need to win a race against a 100-year-old man?

A decade ago, Greg Glassman predicted CrossFitters would someday deadlift 600lbs, run a sub-six-minute mile and perform an Iron Cross on the same day. He was mocked. In fact, he was accused of wasting the time of his clients: "You'll never achieve all three at once! It's ridiculous! And you'll injure everyone if you try!"

Last year, Sam Dancer pulled 630lbs at the Games.

Then he ran a sub-six-minute mile. Next, he did some muscle-ups.

This week, I've seen two other CrossFitters deadlift over 600lbs just in my Facebook feed.

A 600lb deadlift isn't just huge for a CrossFitter. It's huge for a powerlifter (I used to be one.) A 370lb clean and jerk is big for a weightlifter, but some CrossFit athletes can do it. CrossFitters are leaner, faster, stronger and fitter than any client at a Globo-gym.

So why are we letting the Globo-gyms make all the money? Because we're scared of what we don't understand. And the solution to fear is education. So let's get started.

Defining Your Perfect Day

Your definition of "wealth" will differ from mine. How much money do you need to be wealthy?

One of the first exercises I work through with mentoring clients is, "What's your perfect day look like?"

In other words, when your business is delivering exactly what you want it to, how do you spend your time?

It's easy to ask, "How much net revenue do you want to make?" but that's dodging the issue, isn't it?

The issue is really, "What kind of life do you want to live?"

Try it: a year from now, when your business is perfect, what time will you wake up in the morning? Will you open the gym, or would someone else? Would you put your kids on the school bus, have a leisurely coffee, and then cruise to work knowing that your early classes went just as well as if you'd delivered them? Would you go to the gym at all, or take a day off on the spur of the moment?

When you got there, would you coach? Would you jump into a group as an athlete? Would you work on further developing the business? Would you take your wife out for lunch? Would you leave early? Would you come back again later, or not?

Some of my clients LOVE to coach, and would prefer that the business run itself. Others would like to learn more about the business side, and cut back on coaching a little. Both are great. The point is: you'll have the choice.

How many vacations would you take each year? Where would you go?

Now: how much net revenue would it take to support this lifestyle? What kind of staff will we need, and how will we support them?

As you can see, the conversation has only just begun. But it's important to start talking about the right things right away, because it's possible to build up a ton of momentum and still be headed in the wrong direction.

BONUS: if you have this list in front of you, you'll look at it. When you're having a challenging day, reviewing your 'perfect day' list will put things in perspective: most box gym owners are always at least 3/4 of the way there. In years of mentoring, and thousands of boxes polled, NO box owner has ever said, "I would quit my job."

That's remarkable.

No matter what your "perfect day" scenario includes, achieving this goal will require assets.

What are assets?

Assets are services and products that create more revenue than they cost. The best assets require the least time to service. Some assets will require very minimal time to service and still produce revenue.

Robert Kiyosaki writes extensively about the difference between assets and liabilities in "Second Chance: For Your Money, Your Life and Our World." Most people would consider their house and cars assets; Kiyosaki doesn't, because they don't produce revenues. Both are costs only. Even when your mortgage is covered, says Kiyosaki, your house is still a liability because ongoing costs (insurance, power, paint) don't move you closer to wealth. Yes, housing is a necessary liability for many, but doesn't have to be: owners of small apartment complexes who occupy one unit can actually make money on their housing.

Historically, real estate was the go-to "asset" for most people trying to create revenue with a minimal time requirement. Even Kiyosaki used this method: buy a property with borrowed money, and lease it for slightly more than the cost of the loan. He spells out the process well in "Rich Dad, Poor Dad," so I won't repeat it here.

The modern economy has many more opportunities. But I'd be remiss if I didn't start with the most obvious example for gym owners: buying your building.

In 2014, my total rent and fixed building costs amounted to $4000 per month, not including variable costs like heat and power. The mortgage payment on a new building was about the same, but I had $70,000 in cash as a down payment, so the mortgage payment dropped to $3500 per month.

The gym still pays $4000 per month in rent, but I'm the landlord. The $500 difference is revenue that requires no extra time to earn. And when the mortgage is paid off, all of the $4000 per month will be revenue requiring very little time to earn. The building is slowly becoming a valuable asset instead of a monthly liability.

You can do the same, even if you don't have $70,000 in cash. Leveraging debt is still a simple process in North America, and there are many seminars describing the process (I'll have one available online soon.)

Some consider a 401(k) or other stocks and bonds an asset. And that can be true; some stocks can produce passive income. But fees for financial "advisors," brokerages and taxes eat far more of the potential upside than most purchasers believe.

Another asset is licensing. If you're a CrossFit gym, you pay a licensing fee to HQ. It's a great deal for the affiliate owner (currently at $3000 / year, there's virtually no brand in the world with more bang for the buck. Many affiliates easily get a return of 100x their investment in the brand.) It's a great deal for HQ, because the administration of the brand costs less than the revenues generated. The brand can also be licensed to corporate sponsors like Reebok and Rogue.

I own the trademark on the IgniteGym brand, and have pending trademarks on others. My partner and I license the use of the brand to various IgniteGym affiliates worldwide. Soon, we'll do the same with ConcussionPro and some others. As the brand grows, the revenue generated by the license will be larger than the time required to maintain the brand. There's a lot of work involved, but we're creating a long-term asset.

Online sales through Amazon and EBay are also assets. Those who set up early resale sites (think craigslist.com) recognized the opportunity before anyone else; many are now multimillionaires. This avenue will only continue to grow. In the Information Age, anyone who can sort and make meaningful recommendations has a real opportunity. Where once our economy was based on trust (you knew the grocer personally,) we now trust experts to filter information for us.

For example, my kids own averysbooks.com. It's an online Amazon store; we don't warehouse children's books in our basement (though it appears that way sometimes.)

Averysbooks.com is a simple blog site with a rotating menu of books my kids have read and recommend for other kids. Every week, my son and daughter write a short blog post about what they've been reading, and add that book to the store. They make 4-6% on each sale (which is usually spent on more books.) As the store grows in popularity, it becomes a larger asset. More importantly, it's preparing them for the world they'll likely encounter when they finish high school.

This filtering is a valuable service. If you take one of my kids to a library, they'll love the choice available to them; but many kids will be paralyzed, and fall back on an author they've already read. Kids who don't read often might not know where to start. The opinion of a voracious reader their own age will help them find books they enjoy, and possibly even spark a lifelong love of reading. If I could guide your kid toward a book they'll love, do you care if MY kid makes $0.40 on the purchase? Of course not.

Coaches have adapted to this new economy model too. When I started coaching in 1996, the best coaches were the ones with the most books. We provided access to limited knowledge, and our service was valuable because we were the only ones who had the knowledge. This is no longer the case: now coaches must be FILTERS for knowledge, because everything is online and accessible.

The democratization of knowledge is good for everyone: clients know more, which means coaches must learn more to outpace them. Coaches must also be able to provide context from their experience: deadlifting isn't always the answer to a bad back, and a good coach can instruct the client on timing, load and appropriate intensity.

Some coaches will adopt new techniques faster than others, and become experts earlier. Their expertise is valuable to new coaches.

I was forced to learn hard lessons about business in 2005, long before many small gyms opened. I started blogging about these lessons in 2008, and compiled a few hundred into a 2012 book called "Two-Brain Business." These proved to be valuable lessons for thousands of other gym owners: for the cover price of the book (less than $20,) gym owners could profit from my victories and avoid my very costly mistakes. I had the information first, and found my experience was valuable to others.

The book was first produced to accompany a seminar I was giving in Florida. It had a green cover with a piece of clip art on the front. At the start of 2015, it had sold over 4,000 copies on Amazon and Barnes&Noble.com. My knowledge created a small asset that generates revenue without much time invested.

Your knowledge can be a very valuable asset. Every day, you earn money teaching your knowledge to others. In the old educational model, you were paid a fixed rate per hour or year. Your price was determined by a teachers' union or collective bargaining, and everyone was paid the same rate to deliver the same information.

In the new open-market model, you're paid the value of your teaching. This can vary over time (a lesson in the air squat is very valuable to a new client, but less valuable to a long-time veteran.) It could be an hourly rate (personal training) or fluctuate based on attendance in a group class. In chapter two, we'll calculate the value of your time and start moving you toward higher-value roles. Many long-time coaches are now offering their teaching online (including me.) After coaching for decades, I know which lessons are most valuable to my clients, and can deliver those lessons in video format. This is great for the client (they can learn anytime, and it costs far less) and good for me (I can help more gyms at once) and great for fitness (if we all succeed, more people get fit.) The key is time: after a few months of long days recording videos and writing text, I have an asset requiring little maintenance. Other coaches are discovering ways to deliver their services to a broader audience in less time. I've taken online courses from many of my coaching heroes, and been excited to learn from experts to which I normally wouldn't have access. Every time, the lessons I've taken from the course far exceeded the cost, and I'm happy knowing the expert is making a good living. I want my heroes to ride off into the sunset.

Some people associate wealth with the "rock star" lifestyle. Musicians are a great example of experts who have created assets through technology.

Two hundred years ago, a musician was paid by the gig or the hour. If they didn't show up, they weren't paid. The tradition stretched back to the earliest days of an agrarian/industrial society.

But technology (the gramophone) made it possible to leverage the musician's expertise. Spending an hour recording your music wouldn't create an immediate paycheck, but that music could be sold over and over to audiences beyond your reach. The great experts of music shifted their attention to these assets, pushing the technology forward. By the time I was a kid, most professional musicians were doing live shows only to promote their real assets (albums.)

Of course, there's always room for local bands, whose expertise hasn't reached a level high enough to produce an asset to leverage. But they COULD get there if they invested the time to become expert. You, the fitness professional, have already taken that leap.

Key to all of these assets: they're never a trade of money for time. Many coaches started as personal trainers, making a set hourly rate for showing up and motivating their clients. The best became very busy, and realized the only way to increase their wealth was to increase their net revenue, because their days were full. They simply had no more time to sell. So they started partnering clients.

This created a less expensive option for the client and more net revenue for the coach. Win-win.

As some trainers became even more esteemed, they found a way to coach groups. This was very tough, because it meant developing a model that would improve everyone's fitness. When I started my career, this was considered an unreachable goal-- until Greg Glassman did it. His model is broad, general and inclusive.

The next step to increasing revenue over time was to open a business and allow others to duplicate the same model, collecting a bit of revenue from their time. And then, because the model was so strong, to teach other coaches how to train others and license the CrossFit brand.

This has only been done once on such a large scale, and it changed the fitness industry. Once again, technology has expanded to accommodate the top experts. And your gym has benefited from this model. Many readers of this book are business owners trying to create an asset: a gym that provides a good living and a means to retire. That's good.

Is your fitness practice an asset?

Whether you own a gym, work in a gym or sell training online, your fitness practice must create net revenue. Enough to support your lifestyle, in most cases. We'll talk about an appropriate margin later in this book.

Unfortunately, many are still focused on trading their time for money. They've bought themselves a job. They're focused on becoming better coaches--good--at the expense of becoming better business owners and creating an asset--bad. They're specialists instead of generalists. We'll change that.

What are liabilities?

A liability is anything with a cost (time or money) that doesn't provide a positive return. As mentioned earlier, your house is not an asset because it doesn't improve your cash flow. It's a liability. Your car probably isn't an asset, and your TV definitely isn't an asset.

In your gym, equipment is likely an asset because it makes your practice possible. Space can be an asset or a liability, depending on the way it's used. Unused space is a liability; the asset value of much-used space is higher than lesser-used space. Bigger isn't better.

Obviously, there's a spectrum of asset value. The value of an asset goes up as the time required to leverage its worth goes down. Your landlord has an asset: you're paying rent every month, and probably don't see him every day. That's a large asset. If your gym business nets you $1 per year, that's a small asset. If it takes you 18 hours/day to reach that $1 net per year, it's a liability, because you could earn more elsewhere.

Is your fitness practice an asset? How big an asset? How big SHOULD it be?

Whether you own a gym, work in a gym or sell training online, your fitness practice must create net revenue. Enough to support your lifestyle, in most cases. We'll talk about an appropriate margin later in this book.

If wealth is net revenue over time, then increasing the value of your time means increasing your wealth. Unfortunately, many are still focused on trading their time for money. They've bought themselves a job. They're focused on becoming better coaches--good--at the expense of becoming better business owners and creating an asset--bad. They're specialists instead of generalists. They focus on "what" instead of "why."

Starting with "Why" Instead of "What"

It should be no surprise that I'm a fan of Simon Sinek's "Start With Why." I don't believe in starting a business just to "buy a job." I believe in the "Authentic Swing," in the words of Steven Pressfield. I believe in practice, and sharpening the sword, but I also believe a business will be an extension of your personality. For a very brief period in 2013, I was cc'd on affiliate applications at CrossFit HQ. My job was to seek out special stories among new affiliate owners and write about them. My inbox was soon overwhelmed, and I couldn't read them all, but there was a strong common theme: "I'm opening this gym because I want to help people."

Almost two years later, I led a survey of 1300 affiliates to take the temperature of the community, and also to find the places where I could help most. I asked the same questions I've been asking myself since 2005: where am I now? Where am I going? If I had it to do all over again, would I?

Not every owner said they'd open a business again if given the chance to go back in time. But EVERY owner said they would spend part of their "perfect day" coaching. That's remarkable. Since writing a summary of the survey data in January, I've been trying to find another occupation where more than HALF the practitioners would turn up for work the day after winning the lottery. I can't find a single one.

Though not every business will thrive (and some, sadly, won't survive,) every gym owner I know started with a desire to help. Their methods might differ; some might be a bit too rough, and others a bit too soft. But they ALL want to help someone.

For a moment, wipe your mental slate clean. Pretend you're the first garage gym in the world. Knowing what you now do about target markets and coaching, who can you help MOST? Who do you want to work with? What's your coaching style? WHY are you in this?

Write that down. Post it on your blog. Tell your story early and often; help people to know you before they meet you. Then be authentic to your coaching style: know your strengths and strategic advantages.

Over the last five years, I've used my gym to host several related services, like IgniteGym.com; ConcussionPro.com; and Spark Rehab. But because my "why" is to improve lives and increase joy in my clients, I've also been able to offer drama groups; creative writing lessons; CampFire Guitar classes; and other seemingly-unrelated gym groups. No one asks, "Why are you learning to play guitar at a gym?" Instead, they know we're dedicated to providing education that makes people happier.

Being Authentic

Before Dustin Hoffman was cast in "The Graduate," Robert Redford tried out for the part. The script called for a college-aged loser who would eventually be seduced by Mrs. Robinson, his landlord.

Director Mike Nichols later told *Vanity Fair* he "interviewed hundreds, maybe thousands, of men" for the part. Most thought Redford was a shoo-in. But Nichols wasn't sure.

"I said, 'You can't play it. You can never play a loser." Nichols recalled. "And Redford said, 'What do you mean? Of course I can play a loser.' And I said, 'O.K., have you ever struck out with a girl?' and he said, 'What do you mean?'"

Exactly.

Robert Redford wasn't authentic in the role of a college virgin.

You don't have to work hard to be a better "people person." You just need to be a person.

In "To Sell is Human," Dan Pink introduces a personality style he calls "Ambivert"—a cross between introversion and extroversion. An ambivert is skilled at placing themselves in another person's shoes. The best part: it's a trainable skill.

Faking an empathetic personality never works. It's not sustainable—people will resent you for your fakery. But developing a sixth sense that allows you to perceive a person's mental state is a skill, just like a handstand.

To practice, follow the Feel-Felt-Found strategy. Ask yourself:

1. How would I feel in the same situation?
2. When have I ever felt the same way?
3. What have I found to fix the problem?

For example, many gym owners have never been too deconditioned to do a single pushup. But as obesity rates rise and activity rates plummet, an emerging market of less-than-beginner clients is emerging.

"Less-than-beginner" means they can do less than they could as a child. It means wall pushups, squats to a high box and Bright

Spots aplenty. It means extra care outside the box—daily check-ins, constant feedback, long emails—it's all part of the package. They might require EATING lessons.

Who can best help these people? A woman (or man) who's BEEN there. They need to know their coach has been through the self-doubt, the rubbing thighs, the absolute fear of public pools and beaches.

Likewise, if a football player wants to improve, he's most likely to look for a football player who can help instead of a personal trainer who likes football. His worldview says "football first," and a trainer will have to establish his expertise in training football players to earn trust (in other words, to be seen as "authentic.") Authenticity is earned ONLY through challenge.

If you're a "hard gainer" who's added 30lbs of muscle to a scrawny frame, you have an opportunity to help others who want to do the same.

If you're in a wheelchair, you have the incredible opportunity to help hundreds of thousands of other chaired athletes. My friends Stouty and Angel are doing just that.

In the spring of 2015, I attended a seminar for coaches of Adaptive Athletes at Reebok CrossFit Back Bay. It was a great experience, but the best lesson wasn't on assessment or exercise prescription. The best lesson was on authenticity.

Angel Gonzalez became a wheelchair athlete after sustaining a rare infection while surfing. Now a gym owner, he travels with the Adaptive Athlete crew to many of their weekend seminars.

While in Boston, Angel was introduced to a teenager who had recently sustained a spinal cord injury. The kid was new to the chair, and his parents fussed over him constantly. Angel took the family to a distant corner of the gym to chat.

First, Angel asked the teen if he'd ever used a "sport" chair. Angel has a high-performance chair he uses for CrossFit and his other sports, and it was sitting between him and the teen.

"Go ahead, try it out." Angel offered. The kid demurred, but Angel insisted.

"You've gotta try this thing. Get in the chair, son." Angel is a big Texan athlete and coach. He's used to being obeyed.

So the teen nodded, and his parents rushed over to help. His dad stabilized his wheelchair while his mom moved his feet closer to the sport chair. His younger brother grabbed an arm, prepared to heave him up and out.

But then Angel raised his big hand and said, "Stop." He looked the teenager in the eye.

"YOU get in my chair," he said. "Just you."

"But I CAN'T," the teen answered. Mom nodded.

"I can help him," she said. "I don't mind."

A mother's love, empathy, and guilt—it's powerful. But what Angel said next was even more powerful:

"Stop handicapping your kid," he said softly.

Mom and dad immediately got the picture. She burst into tears; he clenched and unclenched his fists. Angel didn't break eye contact with the teen.

"You're going to want to go on dates. You have to go to college. You're going to want to drive a truck like mine. You going to let Mom drive you around? Dress you? Pick you up when you tip over? Cause you're going to tip over, son. That's how this goes. And YOU gotta get back in that chair."

That was one silent corner of the gym, let me tell you.

And then the kid said, "Okay, let me try." And he tried. He fell down. Mom reached out to help him. Angel waved her off. After almost ten minutes, the teen collapsed back in his chair, sweaty and exhausted.

"THAT is functional fitness, my man." Angel said. "I don't care about midline stability or how much weight you can put overhead. I care about you getting up off the ground, son. THEN we'll talk about getting you a date."

The kid got the message. Mom was crying openly; dad was visibly choked up. Little brother was avoiding eye contact. And the newly-chaired athlete had THAT look: you know, the "hell yeah. Let's get started now!" look.

I couldn't have said those things, because they wouldn't have been authentic. I haven't been there, except for one "seated" workout I performed with Angel that weekend (he smoked me.) Who are your clients? Look at yourself first. What are the challenges you've overcome? What were the greatest hardships in your life? Those are the largest opportunities to help others. The word "crisis" is derived from the Greek word "krisi" (κρίση) which really means "opportunity."

In 2008, facing potential bankruptcy, I couldn't have predicted that my experiences would help thousands of others. But my ability to use "Feel-Felt-Found" to empathize with others means I can help them. They know I'm authentic. Just as you can't get full insight into a chaired athlete's life from reading a book about spinal cord injuries, other business "coaches" who don't own gyms (or have never bounced their own paycheck) struggle to build rapport with owners who are in the trenches every day.

Your authenticity is a huge advantage. You have others, too.

The Entrepreneurial Path

When I'm speaking at a seminar, I like to draw a chart called, "The Career Arc of a Gym Owner." It's a straight line, traveling through distinct phases until it reaches its peak.

The stages are:

Athlete

Aficionado

Coach

Owner

?

Some in the audience immediately point out that my "Career Arc" isn't actually an arc, but a line. And they're right: most attendees at these seminars are so focused on the apex, they don't see the other side of the curve.

There's a progression from athlete to aficionado to coach to owner. The progression feels like a smooth process because there are few barriers, but the stages are really differentiated by a shift in focus.

Athlete: shift focus to exercise

Aficionado: shift focus solely to perfection, competition or progression

Coach: shift focus from self to others' habits, perfection, competition and progression

Owner: shift focus to coaches and the bigger audience waiting for help.

Each level also requires a different skill set. We all know great athletes who aren't great coaches. And many great coaches struggle as owners. They made the jump to ownership to secure a career as a coach; they bought themselves a job. So the "ownership" skill set is never developed. One of the key identifiers of the coach-who-owns-a-business is a constant reference to "...the business side" of their business. If you own the business, there's no longer a "business side" or "back end." Your primary job is no longer to coach; it's to build the business.

The entrepreneur creates career opportunities for coaches. Each of us finds joy in different roles. Coaches who don't enjoy "the business side" should have the opportunity to help where they're happiest (and most effective): as coaches. But many open their own gyms simply because they can, or because they don't see a career horizon any other way.

The Career Arc of a Gym Owner is drawn to illustrate that horizon. When the gym becomes profitable, will the owner stand atop that mountain and look for the next peak, or will they realize they've just bought themselves a job as sherpa?

"Entrepreneur" is an entirely new career. Coaching skills will help, but won't provide all the skills necessary to succeed as Owner.

This new career means starting over, with new mistakes and an entire new education.

Other hallmarks of coaches-who-own-a-business: they believe an excellent service will automatically be successful. They say things like, "I take great care of people and the business takes care of itself," when deep down they KNOW it isn't true. Success isn't automatic, no matter how fantastic the product. This is a very hard lesson--and one of the first for new entrepreneurs.

Here's the good news: hard lessons are the currency of the owner. No good lesson comes cheap. But expensive lessons can be leveraged over and over.

When, in 2008, I realized I had no idea what "cash flow" meant or how to control it, I resisted the urge to study until I was almost bankrupt. I like math, but didn't want to see the black-and-white reality. I didn't want to acknowledge that I had no real plan for success; that I was mostly hoping. I wasted a lot of money doing the wrong things for a long time. But I'll never do those things again, and I can share my experience with thousands of others, saving them tens of thousands of dollars each.

Likewise, small mistakes early in your entrepreneurial career can prevent much larger mistakes later. For example, a bad pricing structure can cost a gym millions of dollars over 20 years. But if an owner has a clear sense of his numbers, makes changes and measures the effect, the difference can be astronomical. Time compounds mistakes AND successes.

Exposure to the ups and downs of business can also make an entrepreneur's life less stressful. "Angel" investors in startups can be calm about failures if their portfolio includes a few successes. Slow traffic in the gym causes lost sleep for a novice owner, but a veteran knows what to do: walk backward through their tracking metrics, find the obstacle and remove it. These strategies can be duplicated over and over. Some of my own mistakes have been so large, they've exceeded the margins of the gym industry, and I can use them to help others in completely different services.

If I have one advantage, it's the ability to make mistakes faster than anyone else. It's almost a superpower. But I let myself make mistakes, because I know I won't make the same one again, and I can save thousands of others from making the SAME mistake. Every mistake has value. Wasting $100 on advertising in Year One can save you thousands later (see "Bullets and Cannonballs" in Two-Brain Business.)

If some of the concepts in this book seem ethereal, or wealth seems too far away to consider now, that's okay. Simple awareness of the goal will keep you moving in the right direction, even if not in a straight line. You need to think about retiring someday, but it doesn't have to be today. I'm 39 and mostly retired. It took almost a decade. You can do it faster or slower—I just hope you do it eventually.

Being The Meta

You can't be all things to everyone. But you can provide access to everything.

In "Help First," I'll tell you how to be seen as the local health and fitness expert. People will knock on your door to ask, "What should I do to solve this problem?" And if you have the solution, you'll both profit. You don't have to BE the solution; you just have to know the answer.

As a new gym owner, this concept was a struggle for me. I believed I had to know more about running than any runner; more about anatomy than any doctor; and more about weightlifting than any lifter. It didn't matter if they were faster, smarter or stronger; I felt I had to establish myself as THE local expert. This self-centered focus put me in competition with those who should have been my collaborators. For years, I battled viciously with those who really weren't my enemies.

Then a running coach asked me for work.

Though hesitant to share my tiny spot of "high ground," I gave her access to my clients. I gave them a chance to run with her. Other runners came to my gym and started lifting weights. Though I knew far more about the science of running, she was more authentic: she could run long, or fast, or long and fast. She was one of them.

I gave myself permission to stop being a "running expert." That was a huge relief.

Next, a bike racer from a local bike store told me he couldn't afford my gym. I asked if he'd like to host an indoor cycling group for the winter. The idea hadn't occurred to him before, but he jumped on it. His classes filled. I made some income, he earned a bit more, and I felt okay about no longer being an expert on cycling.

The same happened with other sports. Then a kids' program. Then a friend wanted to start a Jiu-Jitsu academy, and another wanted to help kids with autism. When we launched those companies, another friend had the idea to start an assistance service to help outside the gym. Lessons learned from one company helped the next company reach success faster.

Meanwhile, I was pulling together the lessons from various business experts and publishing them on DontBuyAds.com. They were written through the lens of experience: I was connecting the dots between education and my own practice. I was connecting the theories of psychologists, behaviorists and marketers. DontBuyAds became the metasource for gym owners: they didn't have to read the books I had read to get the message.

As IgniteGym grew, it became the metaconnector for CrossFit-style training and cognitive research. We weren't doing research, but putting it into practice in a gym and publishing the results. We linked teachers with coaches and psychologists and therapists.

The point is not that we were the experts in every case, but the connector between points of expertise. Alone, an avid cyclist can't build an audience, buy indoor bike trainers, rent space, get insurance and start a cycling group in only seven days. But through my connection to space, insurance and audience, he can.

Dell doesn't build computer parts. Wal-Mart doesn't bottle pickles. They're both metaconnectors. Dell coordinates the assembly of parts; Wal-Mart puts pickles under the same roof as underwear. YOU can be the metaconnector. In the "cobranding" section of "Help First," you'll read a point-by-point explanation of starting a cross referral strategy with other local businesses. When a client wants weight loss, they should be able to find all parts of the puzzle--from nutrition to exercise to clothing alteration--through your guidance. You don't have to be the expert in each case, but everyone can profit when you provide simple connections.

As online learning develops into a viable platform for coaching, more and more coaches are moving their practice online. Three mentoring clients have actually closed down their gyms to teach a broader audience, much larger than any brick and mortar space could hold. My job is to help them connect with their audience in the best possible way; to deliver the most value to the most people.

When I launched the Two-Brain Business mentoring program, I knew I could connect experts with gym owners directly. Until that point, I was the sole conduit between a huge volume of knowledge and the gym business. Now the Academy gives experts a platform: they can create a course and make it available to gym owners, who can choose which courses will help them most. IgniteGym is doing the same, by putting chess champions, memory champions, coaches and some of the best teachers in the world on one platform. Two-Brain Coaching is already starting to link some of the best coaches in the world with other eager coaches who want to learn but can't find the best sources. Gym owners can chat with programmers and select the programming they feel best suits their gym; they can watch free videos from experts; and they can even let our coaches train their coaches. Everyone profits. My role is "connector."

How did I get to be a Metaconnector?

Authenticity. I'm a gym owner, and a coach, and an athlete. People trust their own.

My "Why." People know I'm here to help; HOW I help is less relevant than my intent. After almost 700 free blog posts, hours and hours of video and podcast content, my audience knows that I care more about helping than I do about making money.

I think the only way to save the health of my nation is through fitness. And the only way to save the nation itself is through entrepreneurship: the pursuit of hard innovation.

I got to wealth by working WITH others, not AGAINST others.

The internet doesn't know a single thing. It doesn't have an answer. Neither does Google or Apple. They're access points to everything; they're the Meta version.

Productizing Your Service

An emerging trend in the service industry is to "productize" your service--to create reproducibility in order to drive costs down and increase volume.

The easiest example: instead of delivering the same lecture ten times for $100 each time, a teacher could record his lecture once and sell it a hundred times for $10, netting the same revenue for 1/10th the work. Kim Ki-hoon, an English teacher in South Korea, does this very thing; his net income in 2014 was over 4 million dollars, according to the Wall Street Journal.

When a service is delivered precisely the same way every time, and the content doesn't vary from client to client, technology can open huge doors. However, most services can't be "productized," because not everyone wants the same haircut. Not everyone likes his steak rare.

In cases where a middle ground, or "very good" can be found; where a set of general rules can broadly apply to most clients; where those rules can be taught, with perhaps a small bit of customization, a service CAN be turned into a product.

In my own practice, after working one-on-one with over 600 gym owners, I've found that everyone can benefit from a basic curriculum. I make this available in the Two-Brain Business mentoring program. Then, because every gym has its own unique fingerprint, I include a few one-on-one calls to tailor the program to their specific needs.

While one-on-one attention is critical to success, the combination of video and personal teaching creates the opportunity to deliver my consulting to more gyms at a lower price. I can help more people. Some still prefer one-on-one guidance through the whole process, and that's fine; but for the more adventurous do-it-yourself entrepreneur, I can allow them to progress at their own pace outside of my schedule, and then help when they become stuck. It's a great way to build momentum, and I love it: when I get a client on the phone, they're energized and excited by successful changes they've already made.

There are other opportunities in the service industry (for example, a financial planner could send out a series of videos guiding clients toward different options for life insurance, retirement savings, etc.) but care should be taken: there's no such thing as a one-size-fits-all for most of your clients. Math lessons are the same for everyone (rightly or wrongly, but that's a different story.) History lessons don't change. If I can explain physics more simply than someone else, my videos are worth something. Clients can learn how to apply lipstick, but not cut their own hair. If you productize a system completely, it can't provide a perfect solution.

Another warning: turning your service completely into a product opens the door for commodity pricing. When two products are the same, they compete on price. Services are differentiated by the quality of their provider (value instead of price.)

In the fitness world, CrossFit gyms struggle with this concept: CrossFit is "broad, inclusive fitness," and many coaches try to solve every client's problems with one exercise prescription.

And CrossFit can build a very high level of GPP, which is all most people need. Humans should train to be generalists. But no one thinks about the "whole": they think about themselves and their immediate needs. They think about "thigh gap" and other "trouble areas," and wonder how CrossFit will cure their cellulite. New clients don't think about what I think about: moving better, being stronger. They see "general," and that's the problem.

Consider these statistics:
70% of students believe they have above-average leadership skills.
In ability to get along with others, 85% put themselves above the median; 25% rated themselves in the top 1%.
93% of US citizens believe they're better-than-average drivers.
Most people will claim they have healthier habits than their peers (exercise and eating,) and therefore will also report being healthier than average.

The phenomenon even has a name: illusory superiority. You could call it the "above average effect": people believe they have abnormal needs, because they're above average. We all think we're unique; and we are.

Applied to a group fitness class, illusory superiority means most of your clients consider themselves better than average. That means they have skills and aspirations not shared by everyone else. They don't want conformity or sameness, and if they perceive you're selling only a non-custom, non-special model, they'll look for change eventually. Sadly, it's easy to find derogatory remarks from owners about clients "who think they're unique and special snowflakes." We -- me, you and your clients --are unique. Delivering only one option—"Come to class and do this workout!"-- and turning your fitness coaching service into a product opens the door to commoditization. If all else is equal in the mind of the client, price will be the differentiator.

Worse, the "group class only" model has a high time cost relative to its revenue. Many gyms will have two or three well-attended classes, in which the cost of delivery is low compared to the revenue received. That's the goal. But they'll also have multiple class times that aren't well-attended. Sometimes, these classes are led by coaches who are paid more than the class generates in revenue. Other times, the class is led by an unpaid coach. Usually, the "quieter" classes are taught by the owner for a very low hourly rate.

In the worst cases, busier class times must be "capped" for safety, blocking clients from attending their preferred spot. How long will a person pay for a gym membership they can't use, especially with another gym around the corner?

The scalability of this model is very weak. More revenue depends on more subscribers, which is the goal of "productizing" a service. But in the fitness industry, more subscribers means more coaches, more equipment, more space, more insurance, more risk. And if rates are too low, adding coaches further decreases the profit margin. Sadly, this means more work for less money by many owners --the opposite to "wealth."

The group-only model is also fragile: if a large number of clients leave in a given month, the business can quickly find itself in a downward spiral. Fixed costs don't decrease when a client leaves; coaches are still paid the same when a class goes from profitable to unprofitable. When the 5am class drops from eight attendees to three, the owner still runs the class even though the net is a negative. And as with any commodity, turnover will be high; these gyms fight a revolving door that has them constantly looking for new ways to recruit clients.

Do you want to spend the next 30 years marketing, or coaching? Does your "perfect day" include 12 hours of work, an exhausted and distracted conversation with your wife and seeing your kids only when they're asleep?

After five years as a gym owner, I had the epiphany that nothing would change unless I did. That scared me, and fear is a powerful tool. Rather than wait for things to improve on their own, I embraced change because I really had nothing to lose except the relative comfort of my rut. I realized that, ultimately, it didn't matter who was responsible if I failed; my kids would suffer even if failure wasn't my fault.

Unfortunately, there wasn't a model I could follow at the time; I had to embrace the unknown. That process led to DontBuyAds.com, and eventually to Two-Brain Business. But only after its publication did I hear the phrase, "Antifragile," and begin to understand how the empowerment of other experts would solidify my business.

Other industries have solved many of the problems currently faced by gym owners. While our daily conversations revolve around bar sleeves and floor cleaners, we lose sense of the gestalt: they don't see the forest for the trees. We buy jerk blocks to help with the PRs of clients who just want to drop a few pounds, feel better and take their shirt off at the beach. We overcomplicate our exercise prescriptions instead of always working to find the simplest answers to problems. Worse, we try to force our solutions onto their problems.

Instead of the question, "How do I get more members?" we need to start asking, "How do I become successful?"

Now that you have a picture of your "Perfect Day," we can use it as Point B and work backward. Point A is our current picture. One-on-one mentoring allows for a precise measurement of every gym. However, for the purposes of this book, we'll use the most accurate snapshot of the micro-gym industry available.

In December 2014, I launched the largest industry survey of microgyms ever. I gathered 1300 responses, and reduced bias by reporting findings to every contributor. We didn't charge for the results, and didn't share them with anyone except those owners who contributed. Two-Brain Business is now the only group capable of reaching affiliate owners on this scale.

The full findings are published in the Appendix of this book, along with some notes.

The Risks of Innovation

There's a lot of knockoff press about our gyms lately.

Words like "dangerous" and "extreme" and "injury" are getting tossed around like…well, like search terms and lead generators.

Many link to other articles and videos–sometimes from the same site–with similar titles to further increase SEO. More eyes on their site means more ad revenue; it doesn't matter whose eyes. The way they're making money isn't obvious, but you're supporting them: you're paying attention.

Fifteen years ago, Mel Siff (author of Supertraining) and I shared a private email exchange. I had jumped to his defense in an online training forum, and then asked him how he put up with the constant attacks on his methods. Supertraining was the largest compendium of accumulated training knowledge on earth at the time, and its many facets provided hundreds of opportunities for critique.

Siff, a true genius, explained that successful people create and share. Critics never really create anything; they just try to find holes in the theories of others. This concept is further explained in a blog post called "Scientists Vs. Technicians" from March 2011.

Creation can mean building on previous innovation, or linking two ideas together. Siff was first trained as a mechanical engineer, and brought that knowledge to weightlifting and martial arts.

Greg Glassman didn't invent the clean. He didn't have to. He recognized its value as a conditioning tool and power-creator. He paired the clean with calisthenics, and made it feel like a game.

Kelly Starrett wasn't first to the Mobility game (Mike Robertson had his "Magnificent Mobility" DVD years before.) But KStarr didn't attack Robertson; he took the concept much further instead.

Every time T-Nation, CNN, or past box program staff write about the #dangers of #CrossFit #WODs, ask: what new concept or knowledge have they added to the world?

When a competitor writes a blog post to counter your own, ask: "Are they showing us something better?"

When another box criticizes your programming, ask: "Are their clients happier than mine?"

As Siff told me, "When you put up a target, you can expect people to start shooting." If you're in their sights, it's because you're in front of them. Keep going.

The bottom line: we're winning. Now what?

Businesses thrive by preparing for opportunity and minimizing losses during challenging times. Hope for the best, but plan for the worst, as the saying goes.

Businesses that are more resilient to challenging times— economic downturns, market crashes or low sales—are sometimes called "robust": they can weather the challenge with minimal losses. But the most popular model in CrossFit gyms – selling group classes – isn't robust. Like a chair built on one leg, they're totally dependent on selling memberships. When anything goes wrong—a coach leaving, a new box opening up, or client drama—the business suffers disproportionately.

As you'll read, the Stratified Model is changing the industry, and positively affecting the lives of millions by providing exercise they LOVE. More than efficacy, more than efficiency, the communities and FUN we've brought to the fitness world will keep people working out for the rest of their lives. We should all be millionaires.

To create an asset that will help build the wealth YOU DESERVE, let's start with a solid foundation.

Building A Robust Business

On a macro level, predictable revenues from multiple streams create a robust income. When one stream slows, the others provide income while the owner makes corrections.

If you own several income properties, and one becomes vacant, the others still provide income. But owning a single rental unit can be disastrous if the tenant leaves. This is called "fragility": the potential for a single event to shatter your income. Many entrepreneurs own several businesses or buildings to buttress against a fragile income stream.

On the level of each individual business, care should also be taken to ensure "robustness"—that the chair has more than one leg. In his book, "Antifragile: Things That Benefit from Disorder," Nassim Nicholas Taleb defines an organism that actually becomes stronger when faced with adversity. A business can be antifragile, but it's an extremely rare occurrence; instead, aiming for robustness means the business can weather all but the most extreme storm.

Unfortunately, most gyms offering group fitness classes (boot camp, Jiu-Jitsu or CrossFit) depend solely on one source of revenue: monthly memberships. This means they're susceptible if the unforeseen happens.

For example, if the gym's computer system is hacked and its membership fees stolen for the month, the owner would face a tough choice: ask clients to pay their fees again, or eat the costs for the month. Many gyms lack the reserves to survive the latter, and would have to consider taking a loan to cover costs. This would make them very susceptible to further attacks.

In 2014, when hurricanes buffeted the Northeastern seaboard, many gyms found themselves buried (literally.) Water damage might not have been covered in their lease, or their insurance; costs to move the sand out of their space might have been prohibitive. Worse, with the gym closed and many of their customers displaced, their revenues disappeared over a weekend. Though insured, some simply couldn't tread water until they were rescued, and were left with loans for equipment that no longer worked.

Now imagine the gym owner also sold his programming online to athletes across the country. Those athletes wouldn't have been bothered by the storm, and would have continued to train. The owner could have survived off the secondary income until he was back on his feet…at which point he'd have a stronger market position with less competition.

These are extreme examples, but catastrophe can strike anytime. My mentoring clients are required to pass the "Hit by a bus" test: if they were hit by a bus on the way to work tomorrow, could the business survive without them?

The Stratified Model

A robust business depends on multiple revenue streams to create a stable base. To review: Fragile = one stream of income. A single crop. A one-legged chair. Susceptible to market forces, client trends and intangibles like "loyalty." Robust = multiple streams of income. Five strands of potatoes. A solid base. When one revenue stream is wiped out, the others grow to fill its place. Antifragile = a system that gains from disorder. "Get a free box of donuts with your gym membership!"

The purpose of the stratified model is to create multiple revenue streams for your gym, create multiple opportunities for your coaches, and constant novelty for your members.

When they begin the mentoring process, most gyms are fragile. If anything went wrong—a coach leaving, a new box opening up, or client drama—the business would suffer disproportionately because their chair has only one leg.

Worse, market pressure has many affiliate owners weakening that single leg by dropping their price. When a box owner has 100 members and is barely breaking even, they're in serious trouble and might not even know it.

I've been blogging about the Stratified Pricing Model since 2010 and it's in my book, Two-Brain Business. But here's how it basically works at the gyms I own:

A client comes in, and we talk. Based on my experience, I recommend a course of action that may or may not include group classes. They have options.

I assign them specific homework. They do the homework during Open Gym time.

After awhile, they find something they like and specialize in that area. For example, some might do a weightlifting class. Some might do CrossFit groups three times each week, and one PT session on Saturday. Others might do the opposite.

An unlimited CrossFit group membership at Catalyst gives the client access to as many CrossFit groups as they can handle. If they'd like to practice a skill, do their homework, meet their friends for some extra fun…that's available for about a dollar/day. If they'd like one-on-one attention to help them get over a plateau, that's available for $40 for a half-hour. If they'd like to spend six weeks focusing on gymnastics, there's a course in January for

$79. And if they'd like nutritional guidance, massage or anything else, it's there for them.

Our revenue model isn't limited to our memberships. A sample graph of our typical revenue streams:

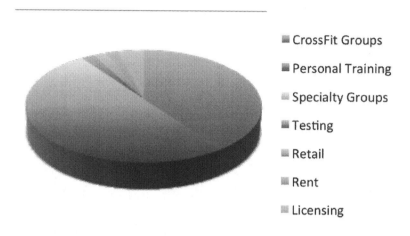

- CrossFit Groups
- Personal Training
- Specialty Groups
- Testing
- Retail
- Rent
- Licensing

This also provides a full-time, meaningful career to our coaches. If forced to live on a flat rate per group, I could only hire part-time people who worked elsewhere. I want full timers committed to their careers; but I don't want to pay salaries, because they're demotivating. The 4/9 model works with the Stratified Model to provide the best opportunities for clients and coaches while stabilizing my business base.

If group sales take a massive hit, it's only a piece of a piece of my business. I can sell CrossFit group classes for less, because I don't depend on them solely for my income; they're part of a self-perpetuating process. I don't worry about losing money in the summer, or over the Christmas holidays, because people put holds on their memberships. I don't have to sell any retail. My retention rate is higher than most, because people don't get bored.

In the past, most of my articles on the Stratified Model were written to convince you, the box owner, to change your strategy. But it's now obvious: the "sell more group memberships!" model doesn't work. Most owners see it, and other "mentors" are now pushing some theoretical variation of the Stratified Model we've been using at Catalyst for almost a decade. That's fine; I want gym owners to have a great business. It's time to focus on what DOES work: building multiple revenue streams that provide a stable base for your business, meaningful careers for your coaches, and a sustainable lifestyle for you. Let's get to work.

"Stacking"

In early 2013, CrossFit Journal sent me to Virginia to meet Joel Salatin. Salatin is a farmer, an author and a great businessman.

At 6am, I drove my rental car across a bumpy track in unmarked farmland to reach Salatin's house. There was no cell reception, so I was trying to juggle my coffee, squint at my notes on a napkin and try to stay on the narrow road. There wasn't another car in sight, and I thought I'd have Salatin all to myself. We'd talk about roosters and "Big Farma" (his term,) and I'd probably be invited to stay for lunch...

That was not to be. Soon after I arrived, his muddy barnyard began to fill with other tourists. By the time we were called to board his "tour"--to hay wagons linked behind a tractor--there were over 100 of us. Did I mention the tour cost $30 each?

Most were at Salatin's farm to learn farming techniques. But my mind was soon snagged on his business model, which he called "stacking."

On his property (600 acres) are several businesses operating together. His own farm sells poultry, beef and ham. His son-in-law rents space for his breeder operation, producing the eggs from whence Salatin's birds come (these are two separate specialties, usually done on different farms.) One of his interns trains livestock dogs; another organizes farm tours like the one I was taking. Others use his space for other purposes, and each feed off the other but exist independently.

"Once you have the land," Salatin said, looking back over his shoulder as he drove the tractor, "You can do anything with it." He was talking about intrapreneurialism in his own way.

Whether you rent your space or own, you can make opportunities for others to build great careers on top. And your brand can serve the same purpose: if you're not currently offering an endurance program, and a coach would like to use your name to build one in exchange for a percentage of gross revenues, you have a potential asset.

If your gym is empty between 9 and 12, and you would rather exercise (or sleep) than take a Personal Training client, why not allow someone else to leverage your brand? The insurance is paid; the lights are on. Create opportunities for "stacking."

How to share the revenue? I recommend the 4/9 model (which I'll cover in great depth in Chapter 6.)

What Are The BEST Gyms Doing?

"Every happy family is the same. But every unhappy family is unhappy in its own way." – Tolstoy

While successful gyms aren't carbon copies of one another, they do have many things in common. Visit some of the most successful gyms and notice what they do. Ask them about their practices behind the scenes. In six years of interaction with hundreds of box gyms, here are the best practices we've noticed in EVERY great gym:

Great gyms:

Lead the warm-up. Start on time, and coach EVERY SECOND. Your clients are paying for your attention, not a boring list on a whiteboard. Make the warm-up engaging, relevant, and different every day.

Are fun. In his speech to Affiliates in Montana last year, Greg Glassman was asked to identify common characteristics among affiliates who DIDN'T make it. His answer was simple: "They're no fun."

Tell them why. You can read about this below.

Create meaningful careers for their coaches. Coaches who are employed full-time, who can control their income, are encouraged to expand themselves through education and have a sense of "Intrapreneurialism" stick around.

Offer personal training. Some things are beyond the scope of a class. Injuries, specific weaknesses, and long-term skill progressions are three. Some clients will love your programming, but won't love the group. Your clients want one-on-one attention; your coaches need it. Give it to them.

Have a low barrier to entry. Affiliates have reached into the living rooms of millions. Some are inspired, but some are scared. Offer a 'step-down' class for people to try. This is different than an "Onramp" program; think of it as a "Lite" version of your classes. Come up with a better name and make it unique.

Look at the whole ocean. 85% of the US population doesn't have a gym membership. Yet.

Can't be easily compared to other gyms. A new member who sees your Unlimited and 3x/week package doesn't know you're a better coach than the next guy. All they know is that you charge more (and maybe have a better haircut?) Take yourself away from commodity pricing. Be different.

These aren't all they're doing. Good branding, great content/SEO, attractive website, long-term planning…these are necessary. But if you're missing anything on the list above, think about it.

Generalists and Specialists

Lately my love for Robert Kiyosaki's books has led me to the writing of R. Buckminster Fuller. In Fuller's "The Wellspring of Reality," he writes about specialists, generalists, survival and extinction. Guess which is best?

We know, thanks to Greg Glassman, that nature abhors the specialist. Fuller's writing predates CrossFit, but centers around the same theme: specialization leads to extinction, generalization to triumph. Specialists know a lot about a little; generalists have a little about a lot. And in general, specialists work for generalists.

In exercise, we know a broad, general and inclusive approach is best for building fitness. You simply can't ignore conditioning work and focus on bench-pressing 700lbs if you want to be fit. Right? However, bench press specialists can ignore fitness to build their bench...for a while. The career span of a competitive bench presser isn't a long one. And we can take the analogy further inside the confines of sport: the more specialized the sport, the shorter the career. Would you agree?

As coaches, we must also be generalists. When we expanded to our box in 2007, I was a competitive powerlifter, and weak in endurance, gymnastics...just about everything else. So I recruited other coaches who were specialists in those areas. A few years ago, realizing we were weak in OLY, we committed to creating specialists in that area. Now we're refocusing on nutrition. While I had a general knowledge of everything, allowing one person to specialize in each means we can go far deeper and create a greater value for our clients.

Business owners, too, must be generalists. Each hat you wear on a daily basis is one area of specialty. These are broken down fully in Two-Brain Business (Roles and Tasks,) but here are some samples:

Coach

Programmer

Bookkeeper

Cleaner

Each of these is distinct from each other, and while I can be moderate at each, someone else will do a better job. They'll care about it more, and if I hand responsibility over to them, it will let me pursue my passion: coaching. Or marketing, or drinking coffee with my feet on my desk.

How do we get there? We clearly spell out the role to be completed. We assign a value to that role, and determine the cost to replace you. Then we spend time in a higher-value role, creating the revenue to pay for the lower-value role. This is the path to freedom.

Moving to Higher-Value Roles

Until you've build systems that make your gym run without you, you don't have a business: you have a pet. And you're wearing the collar!

Here's how to get free:

Clearly define every single role in the business (I break this process down in my book, Two-Brain Business.) Yes, your name might appear beside every one at first. That's fine.

Measure and record how much time is necessary to complete each role every week.

Determine the 'replacement value' of each role – what would it cost to replace you? Can a sixteen-year-old do a better job on social media than you currently are? What's that role worth?

Create opportunities for staff to 'grow up' into each role. This should create more revenue, not cost you more. For example, we group roles together into jobs that will generate more revenue than they cost.

Monitor, track, evaluate.

How closely does the staff person adhere to your checklist, template or instructions? After three months, evaluate their progress. If they're doing well, enjoying their work, and the net revenue created by handing off the position is greater than their pay, you've won: keep going.

Back off. This can be the hard part. As your brain has wired itself to micromanage, it's tough to pull away. However, a good entrepreneur isn't measured by their time investment; a good entrepreneur can replace themselves in their business.

Move to the next role.

Every business has a skill hierarchy. Some roles in your gym simply require a different level of passion and expertise. Some, like "cleaner," are easy to shift to someone else. As you move up the hierarchy toward higher-skill roles, the time required to shift responsibility increases—but you'll move closer to your Perfect Day by large leaps, not small steps.

Example: Came Up From The Bottom

There's a great chance you're not the best cleaner in your gym. Who is? What's a cleaner paid in your area?

For me, $15 per hour is a fair rate for a good cleaner (I know some gyms can't afford to pay their coaches $15 per hour. If you're one of these, scale as necessary.)

If I pay a cleaner for an hour each weeknight, that's $75 per week or about $300 per month. But if I commit to using my "cleaning" time to a higher-value role, I can produce far more than $300 in new revenue for my business.

Hiring a cleaner, in my case, creates 20 hours per month. I can use that time for marketing, development of new programs, improving our Continuing Ed program, creating content, improving my own coaching—or sleeping. Tucking my kids into bed. Eating dinner with my wife.

The rule I make for mentoring clients is this: hire the cleaner. While they're working, move on to the next role until you've produced the revenue to pay the cleaner. Then go home.

The cleaner should be a non-member, if possible. But some gyms will want to trade for membership. If that's the case, write the same contract and checklist for the cleaner, and then subtract the same pay from the value of their membership. That way, there's no grey area: 10 hours of cleaning at a value of $15 is worth $150 in membership fees. If the cleaner did 8 hours this month, they pay the difference. If they did 12, you pay them more. Money was invented for objective measurement of value. Use money to ensure fairness.

Start the cleaner on a three-month contract (when you fire a member-employee, you fire a member.) After three months, evaluate by placing a scale from 1 to 10 on each item in their checklist. Are they reaching 9 or above in all categories? Do they like the work? Are you using the time for CEO work? If yes to all the above, extend the relationship and move to the NEXT role.

For most people, the next most easily leveraged role is social media. Posting to Facebook, Instagram, Twitter and the rest is a simple process that can be broken down into a checklist (I provide my own checklist in "Help First.") The process should take less than two hours every week in total—unless you're sucked into the vortex of Facebook, and wind up losing two hours every DAY watching funny cat videos.

Who is most qualified to make these posts? A teenager with good grammar. In fact, after our Varsity (teen) classes, I'll pass an old phone around and let the KIDS make our Instagram posts.

They're better about Instagram (and far more passionate about it.) What's the Social Media role worth? About $15 per hour, in my gym, or $30 per week. How do I spend the time saved? Planning events. When the events net more than $30 per week, I go home and work on the NEXT role.

In each case, you're working to replace yourself in a lower-value role to make time for higher-value roles.

Low-value roles are filled with high-value people. The "low-value" title refers to their potential to grow your business. A filthy bathroom might limit your growth, but contrary to popular opinion a clean bathroom won't bring you closer to wealth. The best option is to move responsibility to someone else and leverage the time saved.

Kill It or Fill It: Maintaining a Minimum Value for Your Time

One of the major purposes of our 10-Week Mentoring program is to build a lifestyle of choice.

In short, we want box owners to choose whether they go to work in the morning, whether they get to spend time coaching, or growing their business, or neither, or both.

When they reach the point of choice, we give them a challenge: take a 3-day weekend. No contact with the gym. Does the ship stay afloat? What challenges arose? It's a test of our system.

To push you toward high-value roles, one exercise is to find the lowest-value hour of your day. That could be a group with one attendee, or an hour of Open Gym where you're required to be present without making any revenue in return.

When found, you have a choice: fill that hour with a service that builds your gym in one week, or kill it. Get bigger, or go home. The math is below.

First, valuing your time:

During Group Class – take total membership revenue (gross) divided by the number of members you have. Include punch cards if you have them, and all other layers of membership. That's your membership revenue per client. Then calculate the average attendance per month (how many times each client shows up. Most software packages can do this easily.) Divide membership revenue per client by average attendance, and you'll have average revenue per visit.

Look at your class times: which is most sparsely attended? What's the average number of people in the group? Multiply that number by average revenue to calculate your gross for that hour.

Second, compare that number against other services you could provide at that time.

If you have five people in a group class, and you're collecting $8 from each, that's only $40 of revenue in that hour. Could you—or another coach—be offering personal training during that time instead?

Third, execute: either fill the class, or kill it.

If the class is at 10am, and the majority of clients attending are mothers aged 30-45, how can you attract more of the same demographic? You have one week to figure it out.

If you CAN'T figure it out, cut the class and go home.

Mentoring clients who reach higher levels of the program are guided through the process to determine their hourly value. When we decide (together) that their time is worth a minimum of $20, they move lower-value roles and schedules to others. Of course, their infrastructure has been built to withstand the change first...but then they're assigned OTHER roles of higher value. Or just bed rest.

Try it: can you find your lowest-value hour? Can you fill it—or have the guts to kill it?

Tactic: The Nutritional Base

In any box curriculum, the base of the hierarchical pyramid is Nutrition.

Eating comes first – before air squats, before pull-ups, before the Open.

In fact, if our businesses truly followed the ideal of providing results as our main service, we'd be operating nutrition centers with gyms in the back.

Nutrition isn't as exciting as thrusters, but it's important. Unfortunately, there is a great deal of misinformation about nutrition: bad advice is prominent online, in the media, and in our schools. Your clients NEED solid information, delivered daily, with goals, challenges, novelty, and the rest. Just as your clients need to know how to properly execute a squat, they need to know which foods to eat to maximize performance. And yet, few of us provide nutritional guidance as a service to members.

If a Paleo nutritionist said to her client, "Here is the precise menu I'd like you to follow tomorrow. We'll be doing a carb-loading phase next week for competition. We've cut back on your long-chain triglycerides this week, but we'll get back into them in March. By the way, you should do some squats every day…" we'd measure her advice as being incomplete. Isn't this the same as writing detailed programming, and giving a blanket recommendation for more fish oil?

Here are some examples of ways to deliver a nutrition programming service at your Box.

Some clients may need one, many, or all of these to keep them on track, just the way they need a combination of programs, one-on-one attention, and competitions to keep them fit.

- Consultation/Measurement/Discussion of options (Zone, Primal, Paleo, IIFYM, Weight Watchers...)
- Individualized meal plans
- Regular "accountability" sessions (once per month, once biweekly...)
- Recipes and food preparation instructions (free content on your site, usually)
- Private shopping, or grocery coaching
- Access to resources
- Expert guests
- Food support groups
- Events
- Food delivery service (pre-prepared meals.)
- Fresh food delivery (farmer CSAs.)

Each of these is readily available in your community, provided you know where to look.

Your opportunity lies in providing clients access to that information through one portal: your gym.

While it's certainly fine to hold a free monthly nutritional seminar, or post nutrition tips on your website, you will want to charge for nutritional coaching. Sometimes, by offering nutritional advice for free, gyms are doing more harm than good. You can provide a better service, drive more revenue, and help clients more by giving them access to the level of service they require.

Examples:

- Individual Consultation: $70 – one hour of discussion, measurement, 'how-to'
- Personalized Food Plan for 3 months: $150
- Follow-up discussions to keep client on track: $35, 30 minutes, once per month

The best part: someone other than the owner can deliver any of these. A nutritionist, dietitian, Naturopath, or self-made expert with credibility can be granted access to your clientele, and revenues can be shared. Their expertise, plus yours, makes a formidable combination. Again, it's up to you to research who you want to be a part of your team.

The BEST part: your clients benefit.

They are likely to become more informed, more involved, healthier, and, ultimately, happier.

But should all these things be free?

What does your new member want? *That* one: she who just wandered in and is standing awkwardly by the door.

She's never seen this before, never heard of a "thruster," never heard the word "community." She just wants to fit into her embarrassing bathing suit, and hopes you can get her there.

Every website she visited said, "Best coaches! Best programming! Best community!" so she decided to check out the gym closest to her house. You're that gym, and here she is!

Prices are high, but less than she'd pay a personal trainer. She's ready to commit to an "unlimited" membership until she sees the schedule: yoga on Thursday nights. Kickboxing on Tuesdays. Endurance on Wednesdays. But she doesn't want those: how much just to do CrossFit?

They're all "included," you tell her. It's a "perk" you give to your clients to "add value"—even though not every client wants to attend your Monday Night Barbell Club.

She thinks: "Why do I have to pay for things I don't want?" Then she starts thinking about all those other gyms in town…

Instead of adding more classes to your schedule at no extra cost, consider this: charge for CrossFit classes.

Make options available for those who WANT more, and make those services excellent, too. Then charge separately for them.

"But Open Gym has always been free on Sundays…" isn't a good excuse not to improve the service and charge for it. No, members won't pay more for 2 hours of access on Sunday morning. But a comprehensive service with great access and a reason to attend IS worth more.

Readers will recall at CrossFit Catalyst, we tell clients "An unlimited CrossFit membership costs X. You can come to class as often as you like. If you'd like a bit of extra time to practice or play around with your friends; do homework assigned by your coach, or do some extra strength work, it's about a buck a day ($40/month.) If you'd like some one-on-one time with a coach's focused attention, video review and homework, that's $45 for a half hour. Most members do this once or twice each month."

In short: "don't pay for anything you don't want."

For members who DO want more – specialty groups, one-on-one coaching, Open Gym – it's available. When you offer a high-quality service, charge for it. Don't try to lump everything together.

The 10-Hour CEO

Many gym owners are nervous about shifting offstage. They opened their box to be in the spotlight, after all, not to work in the costume department. They see "the business side" as a boring desk job requiring a manager. In other words, the very life they sought to escape when they opened a gym.

As an exercise, draw a picture of a CEO here:

(don't forget his necktie.)
Does your picture involve a briefcase? Suit? Comb over?

None of us want to be that guy. And none of us has to be.

The CEO of your gym is responsible for setting the vision; planning long-term objectives; creating the processes to replace him; finding a replacement. The CEO dreams up new programs and revenue streams, and when they're dialed in, he hands them off to a manager. The CEO tries new marketing, then hands off his idea. The CEO attends meetings, writes contracts, forms partnerships. He's in charge of ideas. Others are in charge of fulfillment.

The CEO role requires 10 hours of work...per month. Even less than Tim Ferris' Four-Hour Workweek. Ferris created streams of revenue (which he called "muses," and I call "assets") and then spent about four hours each week as CEO, watching his systems work on their own.

In your gym, the CEO role will change over time. At first, those 10 hours per month will be spent solidifying your foundation (or simply building one.) The same 10 will eventually be used for creating a pricing structure, and then long-term planning for staff, and then marketing. As those tasks are systemized, the CEO moves on to seek new opportunities: a second location, an event or an entirely different revenue stream.

Ten hours, set aside each month for growing your business, is all it takes. When we start a new client through the mentoring program, those ten hours are usually spent doing the homework I assign. The tasks are more remedial, and involve more math and formality. But those tasks are only done once; you won't need a new staff handbook every month, for example.

As the mentoring client progresses, the same ten hours are set aside for higher-value roles. When those can be passed on, they are. And the ladder effect continues: the gym owner masters each role, then moves to the next, "promoting" herself until she reaches her "perfect day."

The 10 Hours never end. Even with multiple businesses running themselves, I always spend at least 10 hours every month in the CEO chair, pursuing new assets and developing new avenues. I don't smoke a cigar, but it's still fun.

The 10-Hour CEO: A 10-Week Programming Skills Progression

As gym owners, we're used to progressive resistance. We're used to programming workouts with an end in mind. And we're used to having our loads laid out for us. Plan the work, and work the plan.

Many reading this book will see opportunities everywhere and try to implement everything at once. Others will skip ahead to the marketing sections. And far more will become paralyzed by the volume of information here. They'll ask, "But where do I START?!?"

Fair question. One-on-one mentoring, like one-on-one coaching, provides the optimum progression and solution for an individual gym. But gym owners can START with a template. Following the "Good-Better-Best" principle:

Good: Read this book. Follow the template. Get work done.
Better: Gain context on each topic and do BETTER work in the Two-Brain Business mentoring program.
Best: Be guided step by step to optimize results.

Unacceptable: do nothing.

If you finish this book, and haven't made any changes or sought help after seven days, you've wasted money. Ideas without action are wishes. As my grandfather used to tell me, "You can wish in one hand and pee in the other and see which gets full faster."

Momentum is the greatest force in nature. Gravity used to hold that title, until we found a catalyst for explosion and punched through to the moon. So let's start with a little catalyst of our own: a 10-week progression to 10-Hour CEO.

Skills for each week are listed, and broken down in this book as well as "Two-Brain Business" and "Help First."

Time is literal: one hour means precisely one uninterrupted hour. Set a clock (I know you have a big one.) If the task takes longer, stop anyway and restart at the next CEO hour. If the task is too easy, scale up to the next task.

Intensity: don't shoot for perfection. Aim for completion instead. You can always come back later and add a glossy cover. Get words on paper.

Consistency: I recommend scheduling the same time every week for work. Make appointments with yourself. Set alarms. If you "book" an hour into your scheduling software or Google Calendar, be strict: you are your own most important client.

The template below is based on an owner who coaches early morning classes. It's optimized for creative power and processing speed; the important work is front-loaded in the week because stress, fatigue and cognitive load make us less efficient at the end of the week. After almost 20 years of coaching, I don't require the same brainpower to lead a client as I do to think creatively about business. Coaching is relaxing and doesn't fatigue me, no matter how much I'm required to yell or hop up and down to motivate clients.

If this is different from your schedule, that's fine: plug the tasks from your Timeline into your own calendar.

Progressions: "to-do" items are as specific as possible, and follow the general progression from solidifying your business foundation to fixing your retention system to recruiting new members to building assets. But tactics will differ from gym to gym, as will pace and schedule. Make adjustments to workflow as necessary.

Week One: 1 Hour
Complete "Perfect Day" exercise. Start work on Target Market/Services identification worksheet. Schedule staff meeting to review opportunities.

Week	Monday	Tuesday	Wednesday	Thursday	Friday	Saturday	Sunday
6:00 AM	class	class	class	class	class		
7:00 AM	class	class	class	class	class		
8:00 AM	CEO						programming
9:00 AM						class	programming
10:00 AM						class	programming
11:00 AM							
12:00 PM	class	class	class	class	class		
1:00 PM							
2:00 PM							
3:00 PM							
4:00 PM							
5:00 PM	class	class	class	class	class		
6:00 PM	class	class	class	class	class		
7:00 PM	class	class	class	class	class		
8:00 PM	class	class	class	class	class		

Week Two: 2 Hours

Session 1: Identify "low-hanging fruit" on Target Market/Services sheet. Which can be easily implemented with the resources you currently have? Which would your current clients greet with open arms? What changes are necessary to implement? What materials are necessary to prepare for launch?

Session 2: Staff meeting. Outline new opportunities for services and non-coaching roles. Get staff members thinking about possible careers. Brainstorm ideas without formalizing anything. Cue staff on the need for "best practices" and consistency to create the best possible opportunities for them. Note eagerness and prepare to prioritize staff for larger roles.

Week	Monday	Tuesday	Wednesday	Thursday	Friday	Saturday	Sunday
6:00 AM	class	class	class	class	class		
7:00 AM	class	class	class	class	class		
8:00 AM	CEO			CEO			programming
9:00 AM						class	programming
10:00 AM						class	programming
11:00 AM							
12:00 PM	class	class	class	class	class		
1:00 PM							
2:00 PM							
3:00 PM							
4:00 PM							
5:00 PM	class	class	class	class	class		
6:00 PM	class	class	class	class	class		
7:00 PM	class	class	class	class	class		
8:00 PM	class	class	class	class	class		

Week Three: 3 Hours

Session 1: Staff Roles and Tasks. Break down every "hat" you wear into its own role (see the above section on Roles and Tasks.) Shoot for 12-14 roles with 10-12 tasks assigned to each.

Session 2: Use the Roles and Tasks to create job descriptions (just bullet points.) Duplicate these to build contracts for existing staff, and copy the same to create evaluations. Set an evaluation calendar for the next year (one evaluation per role every 3 months.)

Session 3: Create online infrastructure for the top Market/Service opportunity you're not currently doing or optimizing. Walk yourself through the process in reverse: build a clickable "pay now" link in your booking/billing software. Write a blog post outlining the benefits of the service. Assign staff schedules. Launch if ready.

Week	Monday	Tuesday	Wednesday	Thursday	Friday	Saturday	Sunday
6:00 AM	class	class	class	class	class		
7:00 AM	class	class	class	class	class	CEO	
8:00 AM	CEO			CEO			programming
9:00 AM						class	programming
10:00 AM						class	programming
11:00 AM							
12:00 PM	class	class	class	class	class		
1:00 PM							
2:00 PM							
3:00 PM							
4:00 PM							
5:00 PM	class	class	class	class	class		
6:00 PM	class	class	class	class	class		
7:00 PM	class	class	class	class	class		
8:00 PM	class	class	class	class	class		

Week Four: 4 Hours

Session 1: Begin consolidation of "best practices" in your gym. How should a class run, minute-by-minute? How should a PT session be run? Create the simple checklists: opening, closing, and cleaning.

Session 2: Finalize contracts for staff, including role breakdowns. Schedule appointments for review.

Session 3: Invite 2-3 clients to "try out" the first new service you're launching. For example: "Mary, you've been such a great client, and I know you're working hard on those pull-ups. We're about to kick off our new Skill Sessions service, and I really respect your feedback. Would you like to try a 30-minute session on me? We'll focus on getting you closer to that pull-up, and you can tell me how you liked it afterward. OK?"

Session 4: Evaluate staff one-on-one. Schedule the next staff meeting. Provide two choices for meeting time, and let them choose; don't try to work around every schedule. Plan to record the meeting but make it as "mandatory" as possible.

Week	Monday	Tuesday	Wednesday	Thursday	Friday	Saturday	Sunday
6:00 AM	class	class	class	class	class		
7:00 AM	class	class	class	class	class	CEO	
8:00 AM	CEO			CEO		CEO	programming
9:00 AM						class	programming
10:00 AM						class	programming
11:00 AM							
12:00 PM	class	class	class	class	class		
1:00 PM							
2:00 PM							
3:00 PM							
4:00 PM							
5:00 PM	class	class	class	class	class		
6:00 PM	class	class	class	class	class		
7:00 PM	class	class	class	class	class		
8:00 PM	class	class	class	class	class		

Week Five: 5 Hours

Session 1: Download "The Big Sheet" tool from the TwoBrainBusiness.com site. Fill in Fixed Costs (including your own wage) and Variable Revenues (memberships, PT sales, etc.)

Session 2: Staff Evaluations (if necessary.)

Session 3: Client "trial" of new service. Write notes on feedback, execution and price afterward.

Session 4: Start Staff Handbook. Include checklists, sample staff evaluations, best practices, pricing and policies. Download an Incident Report Form from AffiliateGuard.info. Write a "table of contents" as a list of other things to include (this is broken down in Two-Brain Business.)

Session 5: Staff Meeting. Introduce new service and brainstorm others. Highlight bright spots in evaluations. Choose one "point of improvement" across the board for focus over the next month, based on weaknesses illuminated in evaluations. Then introduce one topic for Continuing Ed.
Example: "Guys, we're all very strong at starting classes on time. Great job. This month, we're going to work toward 100% check-ins: every client who attends every class gets checked in. What are the barriers to achieving 100% check-ins?

Next, we're going to be studying macronutrients this month. Here's some material to read to get started..."

Week	Monday	Tuesday	Wednesday	Thursday	Friday	Saturday	Sunday
6:00 AM	class	class	class	class	class		
7:00 AM	class	class	class	class	class	CEO	
8:00 AM	CEO			CEO		CEO	programming
9:00 AM						class	programming
10:00 AM						class	programming
11:00 AM							
12:00 PM	class	class	class	class	class		
1:00 PM							
2:00 PM							
3:00 PM							
4:00 PM							
5:00 PM	class	class	class	class	class		
6:00 PM	class	class	class	class	class		
7:00 PM	class	class	class	class	class		
8:00 PM	class	CEO	class	class	class		

Week Six: 6 Hours

Session 1: Finalize staff handbook. Print.

Session 2: Promotion of "new" service. Write a blog post, and email links to clients who might be interested. Mention on WOD posts, mention in class, put links in newsletters, etc.

Session 3: Cash Flow Forecaster: Calculate ARM and LEG. Forecast improvements to ARM with add-on services (just throw numbers at the wall: "What if one person bought one package of 10 Personal Training sessions every month? What if two people did?") Forecast changes to LEG ("what if we improved our year-over-year retention by 10%? What if we kept people 3 months longer?")

Session 4: Change your intake process. Review "Bright Spots" and write an intake interview / follow-up process. Download my process on twobrainbusiness.com.

Session 5: Work backward through the client's booking process. Build clickable links to your schedule. Post links on every page of your website.

Session 6: Identify your "Joy Girl" (client retention person) and make them an offer for 2 hours' work each week. Write their contract and evaluation form. Start a tracking sheet for calls, broken up by Intake, PRs and Retention calls.

Week	Monday	Tuesday	Wednesday	Thursday	Friday	Saturday	Sunday
6:00 AM	class	class	class	class	class		
7:00 AM	class	class	class	class	class	CEO	
8:00 AM	CEO			CEO		CEO	programming
9:00 AM	CEO					class	programming
10:00 AM						class	programming
11:00 AM							
12:00 PM	class	class	class	class	class		
1:00 PM							
2:00 PM							
3:00 PM							
4:00 PM							
5:00 PM	class	class	class	class	class		
6:00 PM	class	class	class	class	class		
7:00 PM	class	class	class	class	class		
8:00 PM	class	CEO	class	class	class		

Week 7: Seven Hours

Session 1: Identify three Mavens. Send them interview questions, or set up a camera for quick interviews when they're in the gym.

Write down who each Maven lives with, works with and recreates with.

Session 2: Set up a "PR" board and filing system for Bright Spots. Meet with Joy Girl to review the process for calls, emails and texts (pre-write emails and texts.)

Session 3: Identify seasonal highs and lows in revenue history. Which months were highest? Lowest? Begin white boarding specialty groups and events to push weakest months higher.

Session 4: Write your Corporate Intro Letter, and create a Gift Certificate for one free Personal Training session. Leave a blank spot for an expiry date! You'll use these soon.

Session 5: Schedule the next service. Find a specialist that fits your Target Market/Services chart; propose a 4/9 share of gross revenues, and loosely schedule a start date.

Session 6: Sign up for newsletter software. Build a general template. Test-send to yourself.

Session 7: Publish first Client Story, with links to your intake process. Share on social media, tagging the client.

Week	Monday	Tuesday	Wednesday	Thursday	Friday	Saturday	Sunday
6:00 AM	class	class	class	class	class		
7:00 AM	CEO	class	class	class	class	CEO	
8:00 AM	CEO			CEO		CEO	programming
9:00 AM	CEO					class	programming
10:00 AM						class	programming
11:00 AM							
12:00 PM	class	class	class	class	class		
1:00 PM							
2:00 PM							
3:00 PM							
4:00 PM							
5:00 PM	class	class	class	class	class		
6:00 PM	class	class	class	class	class		
7:00 PM	class	class	class	class	class		
8:00 PM	class	CEO	class	class	class		

Week 8: Eight Hours

Session 1: Record revenues and update Cash Flow Calculator. Prepare other reports for bookkeeper.

Session 2: Publish second Maven story, and set up third to auto-publish next week.

Session 3: Break down Average Revenues per Visit. Where are the lowest-value times in your day? How can you bring up that average...or sleep in instead? See the "Fill It or Kill It" section.

Session 4: Approach Mavens with ideas to thank them for helping with your business. Offer to help their spouses, workplaces or friends (one approach per maven.)

Session 5: Execute on each Maven approach. Send corporate intro letters, share gift certificates, schedule a team-building session or training class for the Maven's family, friends or coworkers.

Session 6: Identify three clients who work in the service field: real estate agents, accountants, hairdressers, salesmen...Email each and offer to post their business card on a "referral board" at your gym.

Session 7: Build your first newsletter with Client Stories and links to register for specific services.

Session 8: Staff Meeting. Review staff handbook. Allow room for feedback, but all staff should commit to following it verbatim by the end of the one-hour meeting. Include a signatures page for more psychological buy-in.

Week	Monday	Tuesday	Wednesday	Thursday	Friday	Saturday	Sunday
6:00 AM	CEO	class	class	class	class		
7:00 AM	CEO	class	class	class	class	CEO	
8:00 AM	CEO			CEO		CEO	programming
9:00 AM	CEO						programming
10:00 AM							programming
11:00 AM							
12:00 PM	class	class	class	class	class		
1:00 PM							
2:00 PM							
3:00 PM							
4:00 PM							
5:00 PM	class	class	class	class	class		
6:00 PM	class	class	class	class	class		
7:00 PM	class	class	class	class	class		
8:00 PM	class	CEO	class	class	class		

Week 9: Nine Hours

Session 1: Build a "referral board" and mount it near your front entrance. Post on your blog about it, inviting all clients who are service professionals to pin their card to the board. Reinforce the "community of trust" in your gym.

Session 2: Send your newsletter (to one general group for now.)

Session 3: Brainstorm 3 more Mavens. Ask each for an interview, in person or via email. Start a "Brand Action" tracking sheet to record the clients you highlight.

Session 4: Hire a replacement for yourself in your lowest-value role. Write a 3-month contract, agree on price, and start before next week.

Session 5: Read about our Advanced Theory Course strategy for training coaches. Write down your most influential sources of information. What should a new coach KNOW before standing in front of your clients for the first time?

Session 6: Approach three service industry professionals and offer them "reward" coupons for their clients.

Session 7: Schedule the start of your new Onramp program launch. Break down the curriculum into the number of sessions required.

Session 8: Create pricing for new Onramp program (or duplicate PT prices.) Create clickable links for those who want to jump right in.

Session 9: Begin planning one larger-scale event. For example, a "Murph Challenge," "WOD and Wine," "Corporate Team-Building Challenge" or "Catalyst Games."

Week	Monday	Tuesday	Wednesday	Thursday	Friday	Saturday	Sunday
6:00 AM	CEO		class	class	class		
7:00 AM	CEO		class	class	class	CEO	
8:00 AM	CEO			CEO		CEO	
9:00 AM	CEO						
10:00 AM	CEO						
11:00 AM							
12:00 PM	class	class	class	class	class		
1:00 PM							
2:00 PM							
3:00 PM							
4:00 PM							
5:00 PM	class	class	class	class	class		
6:00 PM	class	class	class	class	class		
7:00 PM	class	class	class	class	class		
8:00 PM	class	CEO	class	class	class		

Week Ten: 10 Hours

Session 1: Plan to remove yourself from the next lower-level role. Enter staffing costs in Cash Flow Calculator. Decide how you'll spend the time in a way to increase total revenues (and wealth.) Schedule a starting date.

Session 2: Pull together equipment to film each movement in your Onramp program. Choose movements in advance. Schedule staff to help, where necessary. Start a YouTube, Vimeo or Wistia channel.

Session 3: Film as many movement demonstrations as possible in 60 minutes.

Session 4: Send three more Corporate Intro Letters.

Session 5: Commit to a date

Session 6: Video editing. Use iMovie or Corel Video Studio Pro (on a PC) or something similar.

Week	Monday	Tuesday	Wednesday	Thursday	Friday	Saturday	Sunday
6:00 AM	CEO		class	class	class		
7:00 AM	CEO		class	class	class	CEO	
8:00 AM	CEO			CEO		CEO	
9:00 AM	CEO			CEO			
10:00 AM	CEO						
11:00 AM							
12:00 PM	class	class	class		class		
1:00 PM							
2:00 PM							
3:00 PM							
4:00 PM							
5:00 PM	class	class	class		class		
6:00 PM	class	class	class		class		
7:00 PM	class	class	class		class		
8:00 PM	class	CEO	class		class		

Week 12: Ten Hours

1. Staff Meeting. Choose one new "area of improvement." Follow the "How To Run A Staff Meeting" section in this book. Assign first pieces of content.

2. Launch new Onramp with an introductory blog post.

3. Create Facebook group for coaches. Link to new Onramp curriculum. Encourage uploads of marketing content.

4. Update your Brand Action worksheet with marketing plans for the month.

5. Update your Cash Flow forecaster with data from the current month.

6. Create an "Onboarding" chart to track client engagement in the Awareness, Desire, Integration and Retention stages.

….and on, always moving forward.

As you'll notice, the plan moves from very basic (building business systems) toward the more complex (seeking opportunities to help more people.) In Two-Brain Business, I wrote about the levels of employees ideal for each role, from analog to binary and all the way to Entrepreneurial. In Week Ten, many initiatives are still being done for the first time, and should be kept as the CEO's responsibilities until they're mastered. For example, when the Corporate approach has been mastered to the point of easy teach ability and replicability, it can be handed off to someone else. The CEO then moves on to the next initiative.

At the ten-week mark, the CEO isn't saving any time; in fact, they're probably spending MORE time than when they started. But shedding roles will create a 1:1 trade for time, and a 1:2 trade for value, at minimum. These are the baby steps toward wealth. They're necessary, and momentum will build rapidly, but they're not the flashiest steps. Luckily, most won't need repeating for at least a decade. My 2010 Staff Handbook is still 90% intact, with a few small changes (mostly to accommodate new technology.)

Another progression most new CEOs notice is a narrowing of staff. If a gym is being coached by six part-timers, each leading two classes per week, it will probably be necessary to move toward a smaller number of highly motivated professionals. These coaches will be building toward a career in fitness, and will be the cornerstone of wealth. In time, some will move up toward partnership in new ventures...but that's a long way from Week Ten.

The ten weeks aren't complete, of course: the CEO still hasn't built a staff training program, or run an event, or even done most of the marketing tactics I teach. But these steps must be completed first, and in a thirty-year business, these ten are negligible for time but hugely productive for activity. Consider this your Onramp: you already know what to do, but the above is a template for learning in the correct order.

Here's my current week:

Week	Monday	Tuesday	Wednesday	Thursday	Friday	Saturday	Sunday
6:00 AM	class	class	Writing	Writing	Writing		Writing
7:00 AM	class	class	Writing	Writing	Writing	Training	Writing
8:00 AM			Writing	Writing	Writing		Writing
9:00 AM						Class	Training
10:00 AM	321Go	321Go	321Go	321Go	321Go		
11:00 AM	321Go	321Go	321Go	321Go	321Go		
12:00 PM	Training	Training		Training	Training		
1:00 PM	321Go	321Go	321Go	321Go	321Go		
2:00 PM	321Go	321Go	321Go	321Go	321Go		
3:00 PM	321Go	321Go	321Go	321Go	321Go		
4:00 PM							
5:00 PM							
6:00 PM							
7:00 PM							
8:00 PM							

My General Manager does every day-to-day task at the gym; I have a managing partner at IgniteGym. Other assets require very little time per month to manage (less than an hour.) "TwoBrain" time is reserved for helping other gym owners. Though my typical day begins at 4am (when I'm most productive,) I end by 5pm and spend the evenings with family or coaching kids' sports.

Other gym time is spent filming or writing content, recording podcasts or chatting with members.

The most important thing in the chart is its flexibility. With enough staff in place, and the revenue to pay them, the weekly schedule is completely plastic. But it changes on MY terms, not every time someone yells, "FIRE!"

Turning Your Hobby Into A Business

Measuring

You manage what you measure. It's a common phrase in business and box gyms alike.

When Greg Glassman wrote his definition of 'Fitness,' he quantified it. He made it possible to objectively measure fitness for the first time. Measuring fitness meant that we could tell if we were becoming more fit than yesterday--or more fit than our friends. We could compete, if we wanted to. We could get better.

If your "Fran" time improves from seven minutes to four, you're becoming more fit. If your deadlift changes from 350lbs to 400lbs, you're becoming more fit. Without tracking these numbers, however--even if only in your head--you'll never know. Measurement is at the core of box programs.

Knowing your annual retention rate is important. Knowing your gross monthly revenues is important; knowing your net is far more important. Knowing the difference is critical.

Failure to measure progress is detrimental to an athlete; failure to measure an athlete makes for a poor coach. Failure to measure your business makes for a poor businessperson. When you open a gym, you're no longer just an athlete/coach; you take on the responsibility for providing a rewarding job for others, and a great place to train for your clients. Without measurement, you can't do either for long.

Finally, lack of objective measurement introduces a subjectivity bias.

Just as a marathoner believes herself fit until asked to lift something heavy, an entrepreneur may consider their business viable until they're required to grow. Or they get sick. Or they sleep in. Or they need to borrow money. Or…

Even the best teachers are learning this lesson. In Scientific American this month, Peter Stokes is quoted on the improvement of teaching methods. "Very, very, very few instructors have a formal education in how to teach," he says. "We do things, and we think they work. But when you start doing scientific measurement, you realize that some of your ways of doing things have no empirical basis."

You may think that your Onramp program is perfect (I've made that mistake, too.) Maybe it is. You may think your programming is fun, that your coaches are the best in the world, and that your burpee penalties aren't causing people to leave.

But if you don't count the number of people who stick around (or some other metric,) how will you know?

Metrics That Matter

We share a common cognitive bias, you and me: we think we know more than we actually do. It's called, "knowledge over attribution," and it goes like this: if I've read a book and learn something new, I tend to believe everyone else has learned the same lesson. That's going to sound odd, but think about this:

The last time your client wore muddy shoes into a gym and walked straight across the floor, you thought to yourself, "Doesn't she KNOW any better?!" And the answer is: "No, she doesn't." We believe she must be acting rudely, because we've learned not to muddy the floors of others' houses and businesses. But she hasn't; we've over attributed that knowledge.

If I know something, I mistakenly assume that everyone else possesses the same knowledge, and get frustrated when they don't. Likewise, it's human to assume that your singular experience is the best of all possible experiences.

For example, when a new gym owner asks for advice on booking/billing software, the responses they get are zealous:

"ZenPlanner is the best!" "MindBody is WAY better!" "Everyone should use Wodify!" I was this way. I thought MBO was the best software in the universe…until I tried FrontDeskHQ, ZP, Wodify, and PushPress. Now I realize there might be strengths and weaknesses to each.

Ask anyone for their strategy on an Open workout, and they'll tell you the absolute-best, can't-fail choice. "You HAVE to do it the way I did it…" like a gambler with a racehorse. But how many other options have they tried? Is their experience really best, or just the best they know?

What works for one affiliate may not work for all. Heck, it shouldn't.

Anyone who tells you "there's only one way" has only learned one way. And anyone who has never made mistakes has nothing to teach you.

In 2010, I had a choice: hire a business mentor outside the fitness world, or follow the lead of other gyms and use a cookie-cutter approach. I was lucky to have access to a fantastic mentor (he worked on some of the corporate turnarounds you read about in business books) and went that route. Now that I see the long-term effects of the "other" choice, I'm glad I went one-on-one with him.

There's a reason I never say, "Do this thing precisely this way. It works for everyone else." That doesn't work for the clean, or the running heel strike, or the retirement plan. Your gym is different than my gym. They can both be awesome, and yet completely different even if they're on the same street.

"None of us is as good as all of us."-Ray Kroc

I work one-on-one with coaches. I've done it with over 100 gyms, and done free consultations with close to 700 others. When a new one asks for help, I'm drawing on those individual back-and-forth conversations. I'm channeling the metadata, aiming the fire hose at the gym owner seeking help. I'm sharing the combined wisdom of the ghost panel: all who have gone before.

To those who offer their opinion online: thank you.

I've certainly been enriched by your experiences, both good and bad. When a new owner (or a vet) asks a question, they always get a wide variety of passionate responses. Like box gym members cheering for the last to finish, owner support for other affiliates is changing the business world.

But the difference between education and advice is data. It's replicability. If you do something the way I've done it, will the result be exactly the same? Of course not. But will it be very close—maybe even a bit better? Yes. Because we measure what works, and what doesn't.

For example, "I got rid of our Onramp classes and everyone loves it," is an unsubstantiated opinion. Does EVERYONE really love it?

If not everyone, do 90% of newcomers love the change? Have they said so? Do they know any alternative? Do they LOVE it, kinda like it, or are tolerating the change? In other words, what else have you tried?

Objective measurement guides our fitness. We're either running 5k faster than ever before, or we're not. We can either deadlift 400lbs, or we can't.

"I ran a free two-week trial and it's the best thing I've ever done." What else have you done?

"The Smolov Squat program is the best!" Compared to what? CrossFit made fitness measurable. Measurement made the first real definition of fitness possible. Opinion without context takes us the other way: toward myth, luck and dogma. There be monsters. Measure everything. Compare. Try it a different way for three months. Measure the effect. Better, or worse?

Below are some key metrics to track. Start there.

It's easy not to track these metrics. I sometimes fall into bouts of laziness where I don't take time to compare numbers. You can guess the outcome: poorer performance in workouts, more lethargy, less strength. The same things happen in your business. Consider these your "macros."

Net Revenue

The most exciting number you'll ever track is your gross revenue. But it's also one of the least important.

As a new business owner, the volume of cash to flow through your business can be overwhelming. From the outside looking in, ten thousand dollars seems like a huge sum, because most have only the context of their paycheck for comparison. This is what stops many would-be owners: a month's rent, at $2000 or more, is probably more than they have in a savings account. So when the business reaches $10,000 per month in revenue, it seems like a huge deal. $20k feels less exciting, because the new entrepreneur has learned that gross revenue is relative. $30k is less so, and though I went out to dinner when I reached $50k gross revenue in a month, I understood the number meant nothing without considering the costs.

What's the difference between a gym grossing $100,000 per month with $90,000 in expenses and a gym with $20,000 per month and $10,000 in expenses? The owner of the second gym is wealthier.

Even with the same NET income, the second gym probably requires far less time to run, leaving the owner free to build his asset. However, the wealthy owner will understand the relationship between gross revenue and net; she will consider gross revenue an irrelevant statistic on its own.

When larger gyms brag of $1 million in annual revenue, but require 8-12 staff to manage 700 clients in a group-only model, it's not healthy; it's a fragile business. The top line is impressive in the way a 1000lb squat is impressive. But when you consider the costs--health, relationships, injuries, missed opportunities--it's no wonder few people choose that goal.

The first Metric That Matters is your NET revenue: the margin left after Fixed Costs and Coaches' pay. The minimum goal here is 33% of gross.

The 4/9 Model for paying coaches will be discussed later, but for now we'll focus on reaching an operating profit of 33%. This means day-to-day profit; your pay comes from this margin, as does new equipment, savings, etc. 33% of gross isn't too aggressive; it's a starting point for an owner/operator service.

22-25% (or 2/9) of your gross revenue should be enough to cover your fixed costs: the unchanging and unavoidable expenses like rent, loan payments and electricity that never go away.

For most box owners, opening a gym is the first time they've owned a business. They see only black and white--expenses and revenues--and as long as the latter is greater than the former, they're happy. But this leads to a huge blind spot in their business.

If Fixed Costs are too high, one of two things has to happen: either the coaches are underpaid or the business is underpaid. You can be sure the landlord won't be underpaid, and the electric company won't be underpaid for long! The money has to come from somewhere.

Coaches will perform to a level commensurate with their opportunity. If they're underpaid, or volunteers, and don't see any opportunity to grow, they'll see no REASON to grow as coaches. Why should they invest in more education--what difference will it make to them? In the worst-case scenario, they'll pursue the only opportunity they see: opening their own gym.

Well aware of this risk, many box owners will choose to pay their coaches over themselves. They're house-poor: a great box, great team...and they can't buy groceries. Who does this help? I went into great emotional depth on this topic in Two-Brain Business, and won't repeat myself here. But it's critical for the business to have a profit margin of at least 33%.

Final note: if a gym offers a discount for spouses, firemen, teachers, babies and German Shepherds, it ALL comes from the profit margin. Your landlord doesn't shave 10% off the rent because you have a box full of firemen. And the firemen are probably in the gym to protect themselves, not to save $10 per month anyway.

Know your net. That could almost be a hashtag. #knowyournet.

ARMs and LEGs

Several times in this book, I state that a six-figure income is possible in a gym with 150 clients. This depends on controlling fixed costs and paying coaches well, as mentioned above. But it also depends on high Average Revenue per Member.

Before you run out and raise your rates, let's consider the bell curve of consumerism:

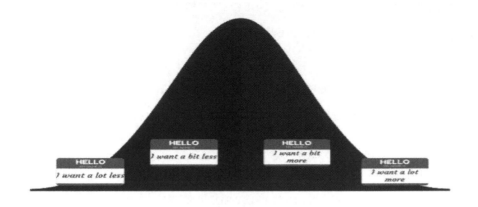

ARM – Average Revenue per Member

If the goal of the gym is to earn a $200 ARM, that doesn't mean every client pays $200 and receives an identical service. Different clients have different needs, after all, and those needs determine the value they ascribe to your service.

If a client prefers privacy to the enthusiasm of a group, the gym should provide an option for privacy. That option will be more expensive, of course.

Let's lay the bell curve over the purchasing habits of 10 clients at Catalyst. As mentioned, clients can pay $135 (currently) for Unlimited CrossFit; they can add as many services as they like for around $40 per month each; or they can choose the 1:1 route, at $40 per session (the package rate.)

Using a cross-section of 10 clients:

3.8 would do at least one 1:1 PT session per month, with an average of 8 PT sessions/month ($320)
5 would do at least one specialty service atop an Unlimited membership ($175)
1.2 would do only the base membership.

Consider the overlaps: if you round up and down, the ARM is actually higher than in this graphic because 3.8 people is really 4 people, and 1.2 is really only one person.
However, here's how this would look on a curve:

The 3.8 people would generate $1216 in gross revenues.
The 5 would generate $875 in gross revenues.
The 1.2 would generate $162 in gross revenues.

Total gross revenue: $225.30

The folks at the left side of the curve are paying only the CrossFit Unlimited rate. For the others, there's no "upsell" required: they just choose the options they like. Catalyst hasn't raised its rates since 2008, and doesn't need to. And the best part: our ARM is actually much higher than in the illustration. High-level clients paying up to $1000/mo aren't reflected in these numbers, and programs like Ignite aren't included either.

LEGs - Length of Engagement

A high ARM is much easier to achieve with long-term clients. A client who has been around for a full year has much more trust in their coach. They're more likely to know where they need more work to round out their fitness, and know where to get the help. Long-term clients increase in value IF you can keep them engaged.

For this reason, retention has been my favorite area of study for over a decade. It's easier to keep a client than to gain a new one, but every athlete's needs change over time. It also helps to consider what brought them to the gym in the first place.

For example, much of CrossFit's appeal in my city is the novelty factor: it's very different from the "fitness" happening up the street at McFitness. When potential clients drive by and see gargantuan tires being flipped by strong women, their eyebrows go up (we've caused at least one fender-bender.) They go home to investigate, and if my website says, "We can solve your problem," they book a No-Sweat Intro session. More than once, a car has screeched to a halt outside and a bewildered cowboy has walked in to ask, *"What the hell is going ON in here?!?"*

There are no car crashes outside McFitness. No tires skidding. We bring these folks in because the novelty of our practice is beyond their scope of reference.

...But after two years, even "constantly varied, functional movement across broad time and modal domains" loses its novelty. "Constantly varied" becomes less so, especially when gyms try to force the Smolov squat cycle on grandmothers.

Later in this book, I'll write about moving clients from subjective to objectively measurable goals. I'll also write about emotional ties vs. logical ties to progress, and how to create all of the above. But for now, let's return to the "novelty" effect.

If, after a year, a client can choose to "specialize" in a gymnastics course for eight weeks, many will do so--just to try something different. Get it? They're DOING something different from everyone else in the world...but not different from what they've been doing for the last 12 months. A change is as good as a rest. But many gyms don't offer a change--do this programming, eat this rare steak, and like it--so the client chooses "rest":

"I'll just take a break for the summer and see how I feel in the fall..."

Specialty groups help with long-term engagement. So do regular Personal Training sessions. But the most important part of client retention is to give them a story.

A story can happen in your gym, of course: Stella can be the one who organizes your Christmas party every year, or participates in the "Yearbook Committee" (see Two-Brain Business) or competes in every event you host. But she can ALSO be the one who was encouraged to run her first 5k, or 10k or marathon by her coach. She can be the one to bike her first 100k or compete in her first weightlifting meet. The point is: long-term clients express their fitness outside the gym. They don't rely on the daily pursuit of PRs and in-gym metrics for motivation at the five-year mark. That's a doomed pursuit.

One of my largest mistakes ever was to alienate a client who started her own group of "running buddies." The client was a fantastic person; she'd made friends in the gym, and invited them all to her place to jog on Sunday mornings. Unfortunately, many of these same people were in my Sunday morning group, and were paying per visit at the time. Also, I needed the money desperately. So I asked her to stop.

She quit. She was right to quit. Others nearly quit, too. Her husband told me (as he was quitting) what a ridiculous mistake I'd made. It was a very painful lesson. They moved away, and he's still doing CrossFit, I hear.

On the other hand, Catalyst has four clients who will reach the 10-year mark in 2015. Others have been around longer (they were Personal Training clients before Catalyst opened in 2005.) The primary difference, aside from the personal attention: I left them alone on weekends, or encouraged them to try new things on their own time. I supported them by turning up to races (or their kids' weddings) but didn't try to force my love of CrossFit on them. To them, it's a tool they use three or four times every week. Finding that balance is the key to increasing Length of Engagement.

LEG is measured in months, but the most impressive metric for retention is YEARS. After all, our goal is to change a person's life;

that won't be accomplished in a six-week boot camp (though change can be initiated in that time!)

Using a system like Bright Spots, a coaching gym should aim for 90% year-over-year retention. That means 9 out of 10 clients who attend on January 1 will attend on December 31.

In contrast, a gym with 95% month-over-month retention is losing 5% of its clientele per month. Over a year, that's a 60% turnover—it means MOST clients who started the year won't finish. That's a huge problem, but it can be addressed.

The worst case is when a gym owner doesn't KNOW his retention rate, and focuses on gaining NEW members instead of keeping the old. With a 60% flow-through rate, he'll spend decades trying to keep people who thought they would like his service…until he gave them a reason not to.

Retention

In 2010, I faced a crisis: some members were asking to cancel their contracts, and I couldn't afford to let them go. But I also hated confrontation; I didn't want to hold them to a contract they didn't want to fulfill; and I knew I was just delaying the inevitable. I started to search for a way to retain clients that was at least as good as a yearlong contract. And I found it.

After speaking with hundreds of gym owners since, I know many feel the same way: they don't want to feel like slimy salespeople or corporate bloodsuckers, but they don't know any other way to keep people around.

The strategy is called "Bright Spots," and we collect data from our own gym and dozens of others to test it. We've been testing it for years, and with small tweaks made over time, I know it's stronger than ANY contract—especially a contract the gym owner won't enforce.

You'll read about the Bright Spots strategy step-by-step in a moment, but for now, let's talk about what your future clients want:

How To Coach Someone In Two Easy Steps
1. Know where they want to go.
2. Tell them how to get there.

Skipping step #1 is silly…and very common.

How Do You Like Your Steak?

"I hope it's rare, because that's how we cook it. And I hope you like it every day, because that's all we serve."

Many gyms now offer a "free trial" as part of their intake process. And that's great, if the client already knows they want to buy.

But if they don't know how your class can solve their problem, or don't know about your expertise first, a free sample won't close the sale. They won't make the connection on their own.

Imagine a new client who wants to lose weight. She doesn't know that your group class is the best way to lose weight. She doesn't know anything about it. Will a "free trial" convince her to call you? Few people will do the research on their own, so for the majority of your target audience the conversation is over before it's begun.

For the few who learn about your service on their own--maybe they visit CrossFit.com, or Google "CrossFit weight loss" and then return to your site--a "free trial" might encourage them to come in. But these are the minority.

Think about the research you do before taking a test-drive: you ask your friends; you think about what your parents drive; you read reviews online. And you already know you need a car to get to work! People looking to get fit know they have to get to point B...but don't know they even need a CAR yet. They know they're hungry, and that you have a restaurant, but don't know anything about your menu. So you sit them down and bring out the bloodiest steak you have.

...and they don't like it. Now what? Do you say, "well, I guess we could cook it a bit more." as an afterthought? Or do you say, "I guess steak just isn't for them?"

Have you ever had a day when you felt like a hamburger instead of a steak?

On May 31, 2015, Greg Glassman gave this statistic: "For every CrossFitter in the world, there are 1750 non-CrossFitters." Do you think they all take their steak rare?

The Client Continuum

The Third Wave

In 2009, it was rare to have a new client walk into the gym. It happened once per week--on a good week. But when they did, I could count on a few things:

1. They'd already visited CrossFit.com, read a bit of the Journal, and knew whom Greg Glassman is.

2. They didn't think they needed coaching.

On one hand, they were prequalified; they knew what they were in for. Many had already "tried CrossFit" in their garage or at the YMCA, and wanted to see "the real thing." On the other, they had already "tried CrossFit" and thought they could do it without a coach. They just wanted to use my bumper plates.

Any new invention attracts customers in waves. First come the early adopters: those who will try something new simply because it's new. They want to be the first with the iPhone 7, or the new game or overhyped car. They want to be different--and they want their friends to KNOW they're different. When I started work at a Personal Training studio in 2000, PT fell into this category; most PT clients wanted 1-on-1 attention so they could talk about their "trainer." CrossFit's early adopters were practitioners who read the website and tried the workouts on their own. Yes, dozens trained with Greg Glassman in Santa Cruz, but they weren't "doing CrossFit"--not yet. He was their "trainer." The early adopters weren't coached, because there weren't any "CrossFit coaches" yet. Almost all chatter between early adopters happened on the CrossFit.com site as comments on posts.

Eventually, many in this first wave of clientele became the first coaches and then the first wave of affiliates.

Most current gym owners fall into the second wave: the "early majority." We saw the early adopters and did what THEY did. We wore the shirts THEY wore, aimed for their "Fran" times. This is a consistent phenomenon with most movements and services. We read the Journal, interacted with others on the CrossFit.com message boards and started to feel our way through the affiliation process. Our first clients were also part of the "early majority," and didn't recognize the need to pay for coaching. After all, our experience wasn't much greater than their own.

Newcomers to my gym today are part of the "third wave"--the late majority. They've heard the word "CrossFit" from a friend or the media, but haven't typically done the research of the second wave. They haven't read the Journal; some believe Rich Froning owns the movement. Many believe affiliates are franchisees. Others believe the opinions posted on CrossFit social media streams reflect the opinion of all affiliates--after all, that's how cults and fitness trends work.

The third wave contains very different clients than the second wave did. The folks who would show up to their first workout wearing an "Infidel" shirt are either gym members or gym owners now. The skull-and-crossbones TypePad blog with the daily WOD as a landing page isn't a turn-on for the third wave. Without doing their own research, this late majority doesn't make the connection between their desired outcomes and our methods. They don't know CrossFit will help them lose weight, or play better basketball.

Luckily, our strategy for attracting these new clients hasn't changed. The tactics are different, but the strategies of telling stories and establishing authority are still there. Doing CrossFit is not a business strategy. Selling CrossFit IS. Look at the CrossFit Facebook page: does our brand list itself as a fitness company? No; we're a media company.

When, in 2009, a new client asked to use the gym without coaching, I had to work hard to establish my authority and demonstrate the value of being coached. In 2015, these clients need the same lesson applied in a different way: they need to know how YOUR service will solve THEIR problem.

The No-Sweat Intro

Training starts with talking.

Your career will depend on your ability to help clients reach their goals. Those goals will change over time, to be sure, but we'd like them to center around your gym.

Selling the same apparent solution to every problem is confusing to the client until you have some context. How can you possibly make a qualified recommendation, or sell your expertise, when you don't know what the client wants? I like to start with that question (and a few others.)

Before any squats, any lunges or even stretching occurs, we want to know a few things about each client:

Who are you?

What do you want?

What are you doing / have you already done?

The answers to these questions will help me recommend the best course of action for the client. Even if I'm going to recommend the SAME course of action for every client, having the conversation first will build trust in my expertise and recommendation:

"After listening to my story, Chris recommended I do CrossFit." Compare this to:

"I went to that CrossFit place, but didn't like it. I'm just looking to lose a bit of weight."

Few of us can afford to make a mistake when people come through the door. Our 20-minute No-Sweat Intro is simply a conversation. I consider the intake process NOT an introduction to any specific ideology or workout, but the start of a behavioral modification plan. To that end, I sought advice from the best behaviorists in the world. Those people don't work in the fitness industry.

In the gym industry, retention (the likelihood a member will still own a membership after a certain period of time) hovers around 43%, according to the sparse data available. Adherence (the likelihood that a member will show up at the gym on a given day) is much worse. The Globogym model encourages low adherence. We don't.

Using the same tricks as Globogyms—free tours or trials, cold calls and free giveaways—might help a future member who already knows they'd like to join. If they've researched your philosophy, then your gym, and then considered their budget and schedule, they're only looking for reasons NOT to sign up. Get out of their way and let them try.

But the broader market, consisting of everyday folks who want to feel better about themselves and maybe shed a few pounds, aren't sure. They aren't sure if your program can help. They aren't sure if they'll fit in. They aren't sure if they really want to risk throwing up in front of strangers. Chances are, if they wouldn't peel off their shirt at the beach to play volleyball with strangers, they'd be better served with a conversation first.

The behavioral modification process doesn't involve a pep talk. There's no sales pitch or lecturing or motivational process at all. Instead, we start with the things a potential client is already doing RIGHT.

We call these things "Bright Spots": positive habits, no matter how small. Bright Spots are habits that can be expanded to block out other habits.

George Lowenstein's "Gap Theory" tells us the closer we are to a particular goal, the more irresistible the goal becomes. This is why you finish a bad novel or stay to the end of a bad movie. But it's also why you don't want to turn around when you're five minutes into a three-hour drive. Anthony Robbins and various motivational speakers call this "momentum." Chip and Dan Heath call it a "20% Bonus." Jim Rohn calls it "the achievement process." Showing a person they're already on the road, instead of just preparing for a trip, will help them get there faster.

Some Bright Spots:

1. "I'm on a diet." – they're paying attention to what they eat.
2. "I have a dog." – they can find an hour to move around after dinner.
3. "I walk to work."
4. "I pack my own lunch."
5. "I jog three or four times every week." – they've already cleared time in their schedule.
6. "I had the guts to walk through your door."

The nature of the Bright Spot doesn't matter. Also of note: the Intro is not the time to debate the merits of different exercise programs or diets. I made this mistake many times in the early days: attempting to impress or demonstrate my expertise through argument.

If I'd simply asked questions and recorded the responses instead of arguing, several of those clients might still be around today. Clients who were greeted with a questioning approach, instead of a confrontational one, stuck around—sometimes for years.

The goal of an Intake interview isn't to turn a train around. It's to put a tiny curve in the track. Let the client build up momentum, change direction slowly, and they'll race ahead.

After three Bright Spots have been determined, the next step is to do a small visualization exercise. Visualization is a science: it takes practice. But we can do a simple exercise with the client to get a better sense of important micro-goals.

If you're a professional coach, you probably already know this: people are bad at setting goals. Their goal-setting process has been skewed toward instant gratification, self-defeat and external "reward."

Goals can be either subjective or objective.

    a) Subjective: "I want to look good."

    b) Objective: "I want to lose 20 pounds."

Objective goals are better because they're measurable. But measurable goals mean nothing without the will to attain them. A person might have one of two reasons for choosing a goal:

    a) Logical: "My doctor said I need to lose 20 pounds."

b) Emotional: "If I lose 20 pounds, I can fit into my tux for my daughter's wedding."

Logical thinking and emotional thinking have been compared to a rider on an elephant. The rider appears to be in charge, but not really; if the elephant has a good reason to bolt, it will. If the rider urges the elephant to turn right, it will—unless it has a reason not to. Maybe it's been a long walk, and the water trough is straight ahead; the elephant won't veer away. Or maybe a FYP (Fine Young Pachyderm) is on the left.

Mary Jane might be "on a diet," but when she's at her sister's wedding, she's going to eat cake. The emotional reasons (celebration, social pressure, cost of the cake) are overwhelming. But if her OWN wedding is in a week's time, and her dress felt tight when she tried it on that morning…she'll skip the cake.

Instead of asking a client to set a goal, have them set a FEELING. Ask how they'll feel.

On her first visit, Mary Jane's goal is to "lose twenty pounds." It's subjective and logical; she probably picked the number almost from the air. She has no emotional attachment to that particular number; it just sounds good. We'd like to move her toward an emotional attachment, at least.

"Mary Jane, let's say I had a magic wand. And let's say I waved the magic wand, and you woke up tomorrow twenty pounds lighter. Without getting on the scale, how will you know the weight is gone?" This question is asked almost verbatim with every weight-loss client.

Mary Jane will likely think about it for a moment, then give you a list that includes:

- "My clothes will feel looser."
- "I'll have more energy."
- "I'll see a difference in the mirror."
- "My husband will notice."

As a professional coach, you'll know that all of these are likely to happen long before she loses twenty pounds, especially if she doesn't have any muscle mass now.

When they DO happen—she notices a bit of space between her tummy and her pants—she'll recall her conversation and think, "Oh, this is what Chris SAID would happen!" Her success will reinforce her faith in her coach and the gym as her plan for success.

Planting these "future bright spots" along the road is a huge motivator.

A few pages ago, I mentioned Lowenstein's Gap Theory: the closer a goal appears, the more irresistible it is. These bright spots, like breadcrumbs along the trail, can provide both short-term future goals and reinforcing "bright spots."

At this point, we've changed the client's goal from logical/subjective to emotional/subjective (from "What will you weigh?" to "How will you feel?") And we can still go further: by creating an emotional attachment to an objectively measurable goal, we can start to use benchmarks, weights and times to retain the client. This is where CrossFit shines beautifully.

To review, the Intake process starts with listening; next comes Bright Spots, and then Future Bright Spots. Finally, we're ready to present our solution to the client's problem.

This next sentence has made hundreds of thousands of dollars for the affiliates under my guidance. It's not a sales pitch, just a question with two possible answers. There's an "A" answer and a "B" answer instead of a "Yes" or "No."

In some cases, the addition of a conversation to the intake process, including this question, has added ten thousand dollars or more in monthly revenue within a few weeks. That's no exaggeration. This question ALONE will usually return the investment in my mentoring program within the first month. Repeated over twenty years, it can create hundreds of thousands of dollars in coaching opportunities that wouldn't otherwise exist. Here's the question:

"Would you feel more comfortable learning to do CrossFit in a small group setting, or would you feel more comfortable learning one-on-one with me?"

It seems almost too simple. But consider the careful selection of emotional cues ("Would you be more comfortable…") emphasis on benefits vs. features ("…learning to do CrossFit…") and peer pressure ("…one-on-one with me?")

I'm don't like to exaggerate. As you'll read later, I despise dogma and drama.

So let's consider some math: a client is curious about your gym, but intimidated by the group environment. Or maybe Mary Jane has read a bogus article about how "unsafe" your philosophy is. In our case, thirty-eight percent of clients choose the one-on-one option over immediate introduction to group training.

Whichever option the client chooses, our first job is to find a physical bright spot. In other words, find something at which the client shines. A point of pride; an accomplishment. Everyone has a particular strength when starting at a new gym. For me, it was deadlifting: I was wrapping up a career as a powerlifter, and had recently pulled a 520lb deadlift in the 198lb class. I was proud of my lifts. So when deadlifting showed up in a workout, you couldn't keep me away. Deadlifting was "my thing."

When a runner comes in to my gym, I don't talk about POSE running, or the value of High-Intensity Intervals over long, slow distance training. I don't say the terms "cardio" or "aerobic base." Instead, I praise them:

"You're already a runner? You're going to really love this workout." Or, "I know you love to run; you're going to kill this!" When a physical or performance Bright Spot has been identified, it can be leveraged to create a Future Bright Spot:

- "Mary Jane, I can't believe you got a double-under on your first day! Amazing. What are you going to do next?"
- "Billy, that's a great row time. Nice work! How fast could you go if you went all-out?"
- "Chris, I can't believe it's your first time deadlifting. You've already deadlifted your bodyweight! Great job. What's your next goal?'

As you can see, we've planted "Future Bright Spots" along the path to lead them. Especially in the early stages of a new behavior, positive feedback is CRITICAL for keeping a client's eyes on the path and feet moving forward. Luckily, in the first days, almost everything a client does is a Personal Best, because they've never done it before. This presents a huge opportunity for a caring coach.

A week after their Intake interview, every client gets a call from one of our coaches (see the "Joy Girl" role.) Their physical Bright Spot is reinforced, and they're asked about Future Bright Spots. "Mary Jane, I heard you were going to attempt three double-unders in a row! Have you done it yet?"

It's only been a week, so success is unlikely. But the client will respond one of three ways:

- "Yes!" – Joy Girl: "Wow, I'm proud of you! What are you going to do next?"
- "Not yet, but I've been coming to class!" – Joy Girl: "Don't worry, we practice double-unders all the time. We're even doing a special jump-rope clinic next month, if you want to come. But stick with it, and I'll see you in class!"
- "No, I don't think this is for Me." – Joy Girl: "That's okay. We think our gym is for everyone, but group training might not be. Would you like to get together one-on-one and work on your double-unders?"

Each of these little goals is an emotional hook into the athlete. One at a time, they're tiny; but when you have many, they're like Velcro. We're slowly moving the client toward objective/emotional goals. We want them to have a strong attachment to measurable progress, and we can reinforce that progress through Personal Records, milestones and podiums. You'll read more about the latter in a moment.

Next, a client is called after every Personal Records. We use an old-fashioned whiteboard to record PRs in every class, but software can sometimes highlight a PR when a member enters her score. At the end of the week, these clients are compiled into a list and called:

"Mary Jane, I saw you had a hundred-pound front squat this week. We're so proud of you! What are you going to do next?" More Bright Spots.

Next to the big question at intake, adding a "Joy Girl" to make these calls is possibly the most important addition a gym can make. When a client goes AWOL, only an emotional attachment can bring them back—and it's not the one most people think. Have you ever been caught by surprise in a breakup? You thought things were fine…but obviously, *they* didn't! This is too often true when we lose a client. We care about them; we invest in them; we tie their success to our self-esteem. When they leave, it's painful. And it doesn't help to call them and say, "Where have you been? We miss you!" because the emotional connection to the gym wasn't really there.

However, the emotional connection to THEIR personal goal was real, and might still be. Reminding them of the goals they set, and allowing them to make the connection between their behavior and their outcome is powerful.

If a client has been absent for two weeks, they get a phone call. It sounds like this:

"Hey, Mary Jane! Hope you're doing well. I'm just calling to ask: are you getting closer to your goal of three double-unders? How about the goal of doing a 5k in under thirty minutes?"

It doesn't work all the time, but it DOES work more than half the time.

The return on this investment—a few minutes' worth of phone calls each week—is one of the best you can make.

A typical phone call is less than five minutes. But the return on the time investment is huge: if the ARM at your gym is $200, for instance, and 50% of the clients come back to the gym after these calls, and you can make 12 in an hour:

$200 X 12 X 50% = $1200 for an hour's work. That's huge.

A client who cancels their membership isn't your enemy. They're the most likely person to join your gym next month…if you handle them correctly. Using a "Bright Spots" call, or inviting them to a free PT session, or even scheduling a goal-setting meeting, can be worth thousands of dollars every year.

Clients don't quit for physical reasons. They give up for psychological reasons. We won't solve the problem without understanding psychology, and that means approaching the problem as a behavioral puzzle to solve. Even when the client cites a logical reason for quitting, like these:

- "I just can't afford it anymore"
- "My schedule changed at work"
- "I just need a break"
- "I'm moving, so my drive will be too long to the gym"

…we can trump them with emotional reasons.

Bright Spots is a simple strategy that will help people stick with exercise—and your gym—for much longer. Some of our clients are reaching the 13-year mark in 2015.

But Bright Spots is just the bare bones of your retention strategy. You'll still need to fill in the gaps between calls and other contact. Every day, a client must see the benefit of being coached.

Onramp, Foundations and Intake Programs

Let us consider the goals of your Onramp program. Here are mine; yours might be different.

First, we want people to learn the basics: how to squat. Where to put their head while pressing. How to use hip extension instead of back extension in the deadlift. How to know the difference.

We'd like our new friends to know a bit about where we're coming from. We want a bit on, "What is fitness?" and a little discussion on Zone, a little on Paleo.

Is our goal to create the best overhead squatter in the Box?

Is our goal proficiency? Consistency? Mastery?

If we're not looking to create perfection in six sessions, then what's our objective?

My answer: to show people that there's more to learn. That's it. I'd like to demonstrate that exercises most take for granted, like the air squat, has skill and nuance that other Coaches don't care about, or don't understand. I'm not looking for a 500lbs back squat in Onramp; I'm trying to get our beginners to show up again on Monday, and again Tuesday, and pursue that heavy back squat over a lifetime.

If your goal is the same, ask yourself: "Does my Onramp curriculum try to address EVERYTHING, and make perfect movers....or does it encourage people to come back and try again?" They're not the same thing.

Onramp shouldn't be the "try before you buy," but the starting point. If your Onramp conversion rate is less than 100%, it requires tweaking.

To keep your clients coming back, you have several tools at your disposal:

- Prequalification. If Onrampers don't know your regular rates before they start Onramp, you're doing them a disservice, and spending brain capital on folks who won't reciprocate. They won't take your investment, in other words, and give you a positive return.
- Bright Spots. Create a rule, right now, that EVERYONE finishes Onramp knowing that they're good at SOMETHING. Give them a win. Double-unders and deadlifts are great.
- 20% Bonus. SHOW people that the hardest part is already

over; that the social hurdle has already been crossed. Integrate your Onrampers into your main classes as a group. Our Onramp program now includes our huge, fun, team-based Saturday morning groups so that the new kids can meet the veterans.

- Gap Theory. Everyone leaves Onramp with a skill they'd like to improve upon. The closer they are to achieving that goal, the more likely they are to stick around for another month. Within that next month, find another goal. Short-term (very short) work best at first, and long-term goals can be added over time.
- Identity. Assign a nickname, a role within the group, a skill-specific identity, or a social responsibility.

Identity examples, in order:

- "Junebug"
- "The Girl Who's Here First"
- "The Burpee Queen"
- "Hey, Junebug. Violet's been having a tough time with the program, and I'm worried she'll drop off when Onramp is done. Can you please make a date with her to show up for her first 'regular' class? I think she just needs to know someone…"
- Daily follow-up emails. It's hard to cram demonstration, trial and a workout into an Onramp session, even when done one-

on-one. Adding information—"What Is Fitness?"—is counterproductive because the client is under stress, under high cognitive load, and doesn't care at that moment. But they WILL care later. Automated emails following each workout will help reinforce the value of your teaching, and give clients shareable content. Their friends are most likely to ask them about CrossFit following their first workout. A shareable link to a Journal article could be at their fingertips at the best time.

For example, after our first session, a Catalyst client receives an automatic email with videos demonstrating the squat and the press (the two movements they practiced that day,) and a link to "Foundations" by Greg Glassman. Hours after the workout, they can read about our philosophy when their brain is ready to process information—and their friends are ready to ask about it. There are more ways to increase retention, but the point is that retention for the LONG term should be the focus of your SHORT-term Onramp programming. No one's a master in a day; keep them coming back to learn the finer points over time.

Tactic: Explaining The "Why"

The key to intake and retention is to consider each person as a unique individual working out with other unique individuals, instead of as part of a group. This is a psychological issue: we tend to pigeonhole groups of people, ascribing the beliefs of one to everyone in the group. For good reason: "Groupthink" is a real phenomenon wherein members of a group DO eventually take on the beliefs of others in the group. But this happens gradually.

If your gym focuses on a group-training model, it's important to address every individual in a group. First, it must be clear how today's workout will benefit them; they won't make that association on their own. "Hard for the sake of hard" will become less exciting eventually. Your job as a coach is to explain WHY a client is doing THIS workout, and why NOW.

As you'll read in "Benefits-Based Programming" later, the most important part of any workout isn't the equipment, but the effect. A quick trip to the whiteboard to explain the benefits of the workout, instead of the features, is critical to retention.

For example:

Part I – Explain the Why

"Today, we'll be doing one of my favorite workouts, called "The Chief." We'll be working very hard for three minutes, and then taking a minute at full-stop rest. This will improve your aerobic capacity by forcing you to work at near-anaerobic threshold levels, and then recovering back to a more sustainable heart rate. But as the workout goes on, recovery will be harder. Choose a weight that will allow you to perform at least five rounds of three power cleans, six pushups and nine air squats in the first interval."

Part II: Predict an Effect

"High-intensity intervals won't just help you with your aerobic capacity, but you'll also burn more fat later, and spare lean muscle tissue. Your metabolism will be cranked up for the rest of the day. In about two hours, you'll be starving, but not dozy. In fact, you'll be ready to punch through a wall to get a donut, so make sure you have some protein and healthy fats packed in your lunch bag."

Part III: Make it Sticky

"A couple of years ago, I was working out with a Games athlete at a small gym in southern California. She was set up right beside me. When I heard "3,2,1...go!" my goal was to keep pace with her for the first round (of five total rounds.) But I saw her get back to the bar so quickly I lost count. Later she told me she had done 8 rounds in the first three-minute interval." Wow.

A full explanation isn't always possible, so I fall back to "Good/Better/Best": Good: Explain the "Why." Every day.
Better: Forecast the effect (you'll be planting Future Bright Spots.)
Best: Share a personal experience or story with the workout.

Tactic: Frequenting The Podium

Every workout presents an opportunity for a "win." If you coach CrossFit, like I do, you have a remarkable opportunity to provide "wins" to people who have never experienced them before. Think about that for a moment. A person with no athletic success can find their first taste of victory at your noon group today.

The key is to have a client define success beforehand, or lay out several different paths to a "win." Not every client is going to do a workout with the weights you've prescribed, or run the full distance, or even finish the workout. That's fine: a finish line should lie just beyond the comfort zone of each client. And this means my finish line will be different from Mary Jane's finish line. How can you best determine a goal for each client in a group? There are two ways:

1. Ask them. "Mary Jane, what will it take to declare a 'win' in this workout?" Using the previous example, she might respond, "Finishing at least three rounds in each three-minute block." Another client might say, "Using the prescribed weight for all five rounds." A veteran might say, "Beating my old record of twenty total rounds."

2. Tell them. There are at least ten ways to win "The Chief":

    *   Use the Rx weight
    *   Perform a minimum number of rounds per interval
    *   Do all the cleans unbroken

- Do all the pushups unbroken
- Do all the air squats unbroken
- Reach a certain number of total rounds
- Maintain a consistent pace of X reps per interval
- Take less than 5 seconds of rest on every transition
- Scale up, or use a harder modification like Atlas stones
- Remain standing afterward

I'm sure you can find more. Laying out these potential "wins" or "podiums" in advance will prepare your clients to find their own Bright Spots in the workout. Ask for their goals in advance. And when they're done, give them the podium. Celebrate their success: write their achievement on a piece of paper or whiteboard. Take their picture beside it. Share it on social media; trumpet their success.

We hold a "podium week" every year. Hundreds of pictures are taken: beaming athletes holding whiteboards with sweaty hands. Their friends see the pictures, ask what the records mean, and praise them. Everyone feels pride.

Tactic: One-On-One Time

Every athlete should get a "win." Every workout should be the best hour of their day. And every client should get one-on-one attention. To reiterate: in a group environment, see ten individuals instead of one group. Set a minimum threshold for coaching each person.

For example, our threshold is 90 seconds of individual time for each person in the group. That's just enough time to watch them squat, give a tip for improvement, and watch them squat again before moving on to the next person.

In large classes, we bring in a second coach if necessary to maintain this minimal threshold. In small classes, the coach will return to the athletes who need guidance most: those struggling, or those close to a PR.

Athletes don't know the threshold; they just know they're receiving specific coaching to improve their performance.

I call this a 'tactic' but it's not optional. It's coaching. Coach individuals in a group, not the group as one unit.

Tactic: Skill Sessions

Just as one-on-one attention is necessary even in a group, an athlete will sometimes benefit most from the focused attention of a coach for longer than 90 seconds. Sometimes, 30 minutes of individual coaching can shave months off a client's journey.

The most obvious example is a high-skill exercise like the muscle-up. In a class setting, where 12 people at different stages of gymnastics are sharing the coach's attention, progress can be slow. If three clients can't do a pull-up, three are working on the dip, three are learning to kip and three are trying to transition, those last three won't get much coaching time. Worse, their challenges in the transition can be wildly different.

Imagine a client named Billy who has been thinking about muscle-ups for three months. Whenever a muscle-up appears in the Workout of the Day, Billy is going to show up at class, savoring that Future Bright Spot and hoping it comes that day.

With a good coach, he'll eventually get a muscle-up. But consider this alternative:

"Billy, you're getting closer every time I see you. If you keep showing up, you'll keep making progress and eventually get that muscle-up. I'm 100% confident you're on the right track.

But if you like, we can get together for a half hour on Tuesday to work on your muscle-up one-on-one. We can focus solely on that movement. I can assess where you are, take a video of your attempts and slow it down for you. Then I can give you some homework to get you to the next step faster. How does that sound?"

If Billy's been attempting a muscle-up for three months, the offer will sound pretty good. The value of progress will usually be worth more than the price of the session, and if it's not, you've already told him he'll get there eventually. If he wants to speed up the process, he can pay a bit more; or not.

It's important to charge for these sessions.

Some gym owners, believing they're "adding value" by allowing clients to stick around after class for some free one-on-one time, are actually undermining their coaching in the group. They're devaluing the membership of clients who CAN'T stay after class, and decreasing their wealth by doing more work for the same money. The free service will use time that could be leveraged for growing the business. And if you give free PT to one client, you can't charge anyone else for it.

Clients paying for group training should get the best possible group experience. But they shouldn't get a one-on-one experience for free; that's a different service, not scalable, and not fair to other clients.

Benefits-Based Programming vs. Features-Based Programming

Early in 2015, I was in Orlando at a "Fuel Your Passion" seminar. One attendee bragged up his box, his coaching and his programming:

"I have everything," he said. "All the toys. We can do anything that pops up at Regionals or the Games. I reinvest every dollar of profit into equipment. We're the only box in Florida with The Pig, I think."

His programming went like this:

"I wrote down a list of every exercise in the L1 handbook, and I make sure we do every one at least once per month. That way I'm following the true 'constantly-varied' model."

Many gym owners believe the same.

But that's not true. A real training model focuses on benefits, not features. Here's the difference:

Benefits-based programming for a cop, ski racer and world-class BJJ competitor:

"Our goal today is to spend 4-7 minutes in an anaerobic state. This will benefit you, Greg, because after you chase down the bad guy you'll need enough energy to fight him. It will help you, Eva, by preparing you for all-out effort on a Super-G. And it will help you, Mike, by keeping you in a high-lactate state for the same duration as your typical match. We'll put you into this anaerobic state with burpee box jumps: you'll hold your breath for a half-second on each jump, spiking your heart rate and requiring a complex motor tasks while in severe oxygen debt."

Features-based programming for the same trio:

"We're going to use the new monkey bars today, and then pull the sleds. We haven't done that in awhile! And then it's time for a Fran retest!"

The latter sounds like a LOT of fun. And it's an exaggeration: I could make the case for including monkey bars, sleds and Fran for cops, ski racers and BJJ athletes. But the former programming model addresses the needs of the client before considering the equipment to be used. This gives newer coaches more flexibility, but MOST importantly, it lets the client know you're writing your programming to best address their goals.

When presented this way, equipment is secondary.

On the business side, many affiliates overspend before they open. They buy OLY platforms, The Worm and curved treadmills for the novelty factor. They believe they have a competitive advantage because they have different toys. But NONE of these are necessary for improved fitness. Worse, their selection probably caters more to the coach's boredom than consideration for their clients. The coach has always wanted an Eleiko bar, so they buy ten for the gym.

This is also true with space: a year ago, many gyms were pursuing the biggest space they could find. This meant industrial space: big warehouses with high ceilings and no neighbors. The goal was to run huge classes without people bumping into one another. But in some cases, this is at odds with what clients wanted: a convenient place to work out (close to their home or workplace) that would provide the results they sought (fat loss or strength) in minimal time. They weren't seeking a 20-minute drive each way to a warehouse where they could get better at CrossFit. When a smaller gym with more personal attention opened a block from their workplace, of COURSE they cancelled their membership at Big Box. They didn't care that the Big Box coach had a Level Four designation, because the Level One trainer at New Box is a lot nicer. And they didn't worry about "the community" at Big Box because they have other friends. And families. And Facebook. All else being equal in the mind of the client, they're going to choose convenience. And they're not wrong to do so.

But if Big Box coaches had explained how each workout was going to help their clients with their 5k instead of their Fran time... Benefits-based programming also solves the equipment-sharing problem. For example, if a gym's programming mandates "Grace" (30 cleans and jerks for time) as the WOD, some coaches struggle with equipment. If the gym is 1500 square feet, and twelve people show up, half will be waiting their "turn" to exercise. Movement standards and rep counting will suffer.

If the gym is larger and 30 people show up, risks increase as the coach's attention is split.

What if 30 people show up for "Grace" in the 1500-square-foot gym?

However, if the goal of the day's programming is to spend 4 to 7 minutes in an uninterrupted anaerobic state, the actual workout prescription is secondary. A high level of lactate can be achieved through cleans and jerks—or with burpee box jumps. Or with burpee pull-ups. Or with shuttle runs.

If the clients understand that your programming is chosen with benefits in mind, they won't mind the change. After all, it's done with their best interests in mind. But if they "train to the test"—if they're doing "Grace" for the sake of "Grace"—they'll be annoyed at the large class size, the wait, and the lack of coaching.

Empowering Others To Fulfill Their Dreams

"You can have anything you want in life IF you can help enough others get what THEY want." – Zig Ziglar

Our gyms offer an opportunity to fulfill a dream – to be our own boss – that many of us have held since our first Lemonade stand. **This notion – of ownership, control, risk and reward – is more important, among those who hold it, than money.** I'll repeat that: the notion of self-fulfillment is more important than money to every new Affiliate I've spoken with in the last six years.

How can you provide these strong feelings of control, entrepreneurialism, and self-actualization to your staff?

How will you keep them in-house, engaged, and wearing your colors long-term?

Through a process I'll call *Intrapreneurialism*.

Intrapreneurialism: allowing your staff to start their own projects under your umbrella.

If you have a new program you'd like to launch, but feel as if you don't have the time or resources, create an opportunity for a staff member to take on the task. Share costs and workload as required, but remember: it's their baby. Let them take as much risk as they're willing to shoulder, and offer them a reward that's in direct proportion to that risk.

The simplest example: adding a Kids program. Almost every Affiliate should have a CFK group, and many have fantastic Coaches who would do well with kids. However, adding CFK creates a lot of work behind the scenes: different streams of programming, scheduling, equipment, and certification…why not offer the project to someone who would like to tackle a large project and see personal reward?

For example, if a staff member takes the CFK certification on their own, creates a schedule and knowledge-based ('expert') content to push the program….their pay for the CFK program will reflect its success. If they're unsuccessful, they'll be paid less. It's not selfish: people WANT it this way. Your share, of course, will be lessened, but the workload will be minimized (and potentially nonexistent, if done properly.)

Benefits to your Coach:

- An opportunity to learn more about something for which they're passionate;
- An opportunity to make more money
- A chance to test out their 'business' smarts
- Self-actualization (satisfaction that they're making a living on THEIR work and brainpower.)

Benefits to you, the Owner:

- Greater retention among Coaching staff
- Less work
- Less risk
- More time

Benefits to the Client (the MOST important part of all):

- A fully-engaged Coach
- New programming
- Consistency at your Box

A final consideration: the risk-reward balance

If your Coach takes a greater risk – perhaps they pay for their new Certification or education, or not; perhaps they purchase new equipment on their own, or not; perhaps they pay rent, or instead make a commission. The greater their risk, the greater the financial reward.

Keep people happy. Let them take the reins.

Show them that they can have a lifelong professional career, and create opportunities for themselves, while still wearing your t-shirt.

Replacing Yourself

Last year, one of our Mentoring clients was trapped by Hurricane Sandy.

Stuck in New Orleans with his head trainer, he was forced to spend three extra days away from his Box.

A month before that, another Mentoring client took his girlfriend away for a 2-day break – his first in several years.

Last month, one of my favorite clients went to Kenya to visit his wife's 107-year-old grandmother. He stayed a few weeks, and his gym was fine without him.

Could you do it?

If you were hit by a bus today, would your Box still open on time tomorrow? Would your classes run the same way if you weren't there? Would your gym family still enjoy the same level of service without your constant presence?

When each of us opened our gyms, we dreamed of the Entrepreneurial lifestyle. We wanted to provide something better: to be the best coach, the best boss, and the best life-changer in the business. NONE of us signed up to be a manager.

Are YOU a manager? How's your schedule these days?
- 5am: Post the WOD. Look for good pictures.
- 5:45am: Open the Doors. Greet people.
- 6am: Coach.
- 7am: Coach.
- 8am: Coach.
- 9am: Call home. Cram food. Drink coffee. Check Facebook. Check voicemail. Check email. Check the main site. Check

the checklist.

- Noon: Coach.
- 1pm: Train – no, wait…put out fires.
- 3pm: Coach.

In our parents' generation, the 'manager' was a coveted position. Wielding a tiny bit of authority, 'manager' ranked between Assistant Manger and Assistant Director. In the decades of IBM-style bureaucracy and workplace hierarchies, 'manager' was a career. Not anymore.

The word, 'manager' has the same root as 'maintenance.' A manager maintains. She doesn't look ahead, and rarely behind; never to the side. A manager allocates, aligns, and does performance reviews. They do not change; they do not grow, except in belt notches.

Question: are you managing? Are you working IN your business, instead of ON your business? Have you bought yourself a JOB?

When we're teaching a clean, it's sometimes tough to get a client to realize that his hips really AREN'T opening all the way up. So we bring out the camera; we take video; we show him where he's wrong; and we say, "…it goes like this."

External proof is sometimes required to force a change in action. If we can objectively measure our performance, we can identify where we must improve. As box members, we'll use the clock to provide that measurement.

Put a stopwatch beside your desk. When you initiate a phone call to a prospective new member, start the clock. When you email a potential client, write your newsletter, post pictures to Facebook, plan your events, sign letters to your mavens….start the clock. Time yourself over the course of a week. Browsing Facebook doesn't count; answering the phone to book appointments doesn't count.

Now, compare that time to your total time spent. Are they equitable?

As owners, we tend to get caught in a rut: show up, coach, eat, coach, and go home. We spend eight, ten, fifteen hours per day DELIVERING the product.

YOU are not the product. Fitness is the product. YOU are the entrepreneur. Your role is to achieve your money, time, and self-fulfillment goals. You can't move forward from the manager's position. The lifeguard does not catch the shark.

A Hierarchy of Staff Qualities

You've found an expert coach.

She's a two-time Olympian. She loves kids, doesn't have high wage expectations, and your clients are excited to meet her.

Then she shows up late, or not at all. Or perhaps she doesn't brush her hair, or talks poorly about clients; maybe she talks poorly about YOU. All of a sudden your expert coach has become a nightmare employee.

When is a great coach not a great employee?

Maslow's **Hierarchy of Needs** describes the order in which necessities for life must be maintained to reach self-actualization (fulfillment.) For coaches to achieve greatness, they cannot neglect the basics.

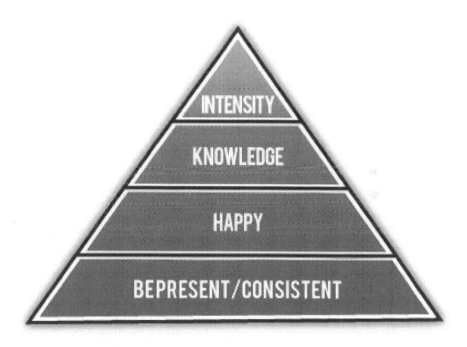

INTENSITY

KNOWLEDGE

HAPPY

BE PRESENT/CONSISTENT

The most important attribute a coach can possess is consistency. While a poorly qualified coach won't engage your members for long, she WILL keep the group running until someone better comes along. Even a mediocre coach can deliver great programming, and if clients are making progress, they'll stay around.

The next most important coaching attribute is, ironically, not coachable. It's happiness. The ability to shelve outside distractions and wear an excited face in front of athletes is critical. It's a non-negotiable skill. Happiness means genuine enthusiasm for your clients at 5am and 9pm, and sometimes both those hours on the same day. Members will come for YEARS to see a happy coach, even when they think they may learn more elsewhere.

A decade ago, a curmudgeonly expert could still make a living, because there weren't many sources of equivalent knowledge. That's no longer the case. Clients won't take time to find your 'soft spot' if you're cranky at 6am. Sadly, many expert coaches with a plethora of knowledge leave the industry because no one likes them.

The third attribute, or level three, is knowledge.

This is usually the first thing we consider in a coach, but shouldn't be. How much does she know? What is her background? A Level One certification is the lowest common denominator: critical, yes, but not enough. Coaching is mentoring, caring about people and wanting to see them succeed. Consider how the coach imparts her experience and passion, how she communicates with others, and how sharing her knowledge motivates your clients. Knowledge can be lost in translation or missed entirely due to a coach's habits. No 'expert' is so exalted that they can show up late in their pajamas. And a great coach who arrives late isn't a coach at all.

Finally, the fourth level is Appropriate Intensity.

Intensity – excitement, passion – driven through knowledge and delivered in a joyous way every time. That's magic. Intensity without knowledge causes injuries; intensity without joy causes fights, and intensity applied inconsistently causes cancelled memberships.

The 4/9 Model

How much should you pay your staff? As much as you can, but not more.

In the service industry, your staff are assets, not liabilities. Every staff person should generate at least twice the revenue they're paid. Keep that figure in mind over the next few sections.

One of the biggest mental roadblocks to success is failing to commit to a profit margin. By nature, many gym owners are anti-corporation, and shy away from any practice that could be perceived by their peers as "big business." Even in 2015, owners are occasionally criticized by other owners for being "too globo," or will comment they're "not in it for the money"---as if that's a bad thing. We're all in it for money. That money can go to groceries, or shoes for our kids or gold watches, but that's our choice. I'll leave the rest for a section called "Failure to Thrive." In the meantime, choosing a set profit margin in advance will help set your prices, pay your coaches and measure your business success.

In the owner-operator service industry, a 33% gross profit margin is pretty average, according to industry data. Globogyms attempt to increase this profit margin through PIF (Paid In Full) client contracts, underpaying staff and productizing their service (everyone follows the same Personal Training and group class template, everyone uses machines.) But we'll start with a 33% operating profit.

Operating profit is your unbound cash flow. It's the money used to pay you; it's the pool for new equipment, usually; it's what covers surprise costs. If we opened on Monday and closed on Tuesday, the money left after paying our bills would be our profit. And we're going to start the process of converting your gym to an asset by setting a 33% profit margin.

Next, we're going to examine our fixed costs: long-term expenses that rarely change. Your rent, insurance, internet fees, loan payments, power bill…these are fixed costs, and our goal is to keep these to 25% of gross revenue or less.

In the 4/9 model, everything left over after covering our fixed costs and protecting our profit margin goes to the coach.

$$1 \quad 1 \quad 1 \quad 1 \quad 1 \quad 1 \quad 1 \quad 1 \quad 1$$

If each dollar is split into nine equal parts, two parts goes to cover fixed costs; three parts to our profit; and the largest share, 4/9, goes to the coaching staff.

How do we increase profit? Not by cutting coaching costs, but by increasing the pie and decreasing fixed costs. As gross revenue grows, our fixed costs stay the same (until we increase our facility size or location, or add more equipment.)

One failure of the "group-only" model, in which the gym owner relies solely on group memberships for revenue, is the imbalance between ratios. More group members mean a higher space requirement, more coaching and more equipment. In striving for a larger pie, many gym owners fail to pay attention to these ratios and sacrifice their margin for short-term growth. This means they're always borrowing: money, for expansion; and time, from their families (or their beds.)

In the 4/9 model, you simply don't grow until your gross revenues warrant growth. Then you take on new debt that will add up to 2/9 or less of your gross revenues.

Do I sometimes jump before the gross revenue is in hand? Of course: that's the nature of entrepreneurialism. But I mitigate that risk with forecasting, and the 4/9 model figures heavily into my forecasts. More on good debt vs. bad debt later.

To recap: in the 4/9 model, gross revenues are split into 9 equal parts. 2 parts should cover your fixed costs. 3/9 should be set aside as profit (or your pay, as owner.) 4/9 should be paid to your coaching staff for their services.

Here's the breakdown for three different services: Personal Training, Specialty Groups and CrossFit groups as performed at Catalyst:

Personal Training:

One Hour PT Session: $70

To the coach (4/9): $31.11

30-Minute PT Session: $45

To the coach (4/9): $20

Specialty Groups:

Barbell Bettys (a strength-specific group for up to 12 women. $89 for 8 weeks, plus $80 for Open Gym access to do homework (if necessary.)

Gross Revenue: $1068

To the coach (4/9): $474.66 (or $59.33 per hour.)

An example in which the coach might not perform every session of the service is CrossFit Kids. We have two CFK coaches.

CrossFit Kids:

Gross Revenue: $3000+ per month

To the coach (4/9): $1333.33

Number of classes per month: 34

Coach is paid per class: $39.21

In each of these examples, the revenue is collected in advance and then paid on delivery.

At Catalyst, we pay 4/9 on every attendee in groups that require a recurring membership (CrossFit.)

To calculate the per-head rate, we take our gross membership revenue and divide by our total membership to derive our Average Revenue per Member (ARM.) Then we divide ARM by Average Visits—the number of times an average client attends in a given month. That will produce Revenue per Visit, to which we apply the 4/9 model.

In our case, that usually means a rate of $4 per head for groups, except for specialty groups (as above.)

Of note: most gyms in our mentoring program adopt the 4/9 model for Personal Training and Specialty groups, but not for CrossFit groups. Changing a pay structure is very tough unless a gym has an intrapreneurial staff person. Unfortunately, fulltime staff is hesitant to jeopardize their salary in return for more potential upside (that's why they're staff, not owners.) And part-time staff don't want risk at all.

In new gyms, the model can be built into the foundation and used very successfully. However, there's an alternative for gyms that don't want to adopt the per-head rate. The alternate is a Stepwise Model.

In a Stepwise model, staff pay is increased depending on a combination of experience and qualification. It's simple; staff know what's required to increase their wage; and it's easy to figure out how to pay a new coach who already has experience.

For example:

Level 1: A new coach, fresh from your internship program, makes $17 per class.

Level 2: After she's coached 100 client hours, her wage is increased to $19.

Level 3: After coaching a further 200 client hours AND attaining an advanced credential, her wage is increased to $21.

Level 4: After coaching a further 300 client hours, and attaining another advanced credential, her wage goes to $23.

…and so on.

When your affiliate grows, and an experienced coach joins your team, how are they paid? Simple: overlay their experience and qualifications onto the above stratification. If they've been coaching for six months but haven't yet earned an advanced credential, they start at $19 per class.

While this system doesn't motivate your staff to be entrepreneurial in the same way as the 4/9 model, it DOES place a high value on continuing education. It could also be combined with the 4/9 model for Personal Training and Specialty Course rates to maximize its effect.

What's most important?

To have a plan for payment, and to share it with your staff. Paying a flat rate per group only reinforces the idea that your coach will have to leave and open her own gym to make a career in the fitness business. Likewise, unscheduled 'raises' based on subjective criteria will break up your team. Any plan is better than none.

As you move from lower-value roles to higher-value roles, you'll be required to place managers in your wake. These aren't necessarily fulltime, salaried men in sweater vests; they just have the responsibility to maintain one area of your business. One role might be that of a "general manager": a staff person good at following instructions, solving day-to-day problems, and performing repetitive tasks. This is the role that ultimately makes your business an asset. When you're not required to answer every email, check in on the cleaning staff or fix the billing software, you're free to expand your current business or start another income stream.

Paying Staff for Other Roles

As mentioned in the "Moving to Higher-Value Roles" section above, some roles in your gym are very leverageable: you can easily replace yourself and reinvest the time into higher-value roles.

In some cases, your coaches might want to adopt non-coaching roles to make extra money or move closer to a fulltime career in fitness. For example, a coach might do a great job in the "Joy Girl" –member management—position. To review the process of hiring and evaluating success:

1. Clearly define the tasks to be done. In my case, the "Joy Girl" calls clients after their No-Sweat Intro; calls them again after they finish Onramp; calls them after every PR; and calls them if they're absent for two weeks. She sends flowers if they're sick and a gift basket when they give birth.

2. Define the time required and value of their service. To me, the process should require about two hours each week and receive $30 in compensation for those two hours.

3. Establish a scale of measurement. If adding a "Joy Girl" role will cost $120 per month, it should generate a minimum of $120 in new revenue. In my case, I prefer each new role to produce at least 2.5x its cost, so my threshold would be $300 in new revenue. I can produce that revenue in the time saved OR, in this case, from the

"new" memberships from members who have dropped off. To be very specific, every client saved from cancellation could count toward the value brought by the Joy Girl role.

4. Establish an evaluation. Add a scale from 1 to 10 for each task listed above. Review their performance after three months, and then decide whether to extend their contract or not.

In some cases, coaches who want to move toward fulltime work can simply add one role at a time until they have a fulltime "job." An example:

Coaching – 20 classes per week

"Joy Girl" – 2 hours per week

Head Coach (programming, staff scheduling, staff training, staff evaluation) -- 4 hours per week

Social Media – 2 hours per week

Marketing (writing the newsletter, creating content, cobranding)– 4 hours per week

Events – 1 hour per week

Admin (entering client data, processing transactions, inventory, ordering supplies) – 8 hours per week

Total: 40 hours.

In most cases, I advise against starting someone from scratch and moving to 40 hours right away. It's best to move up one role at a time. However, this isn't always practical for the gym owner or the staff member.

When hiring someone with multiple roles, it's even MORE critical to have clear contracts, tasks and evaluations in advance. Done one role at a time, there's some room to shift responsibility every three months, depending on need and the strengths of the staff member. Done all at once, things become tougher to measure. I recommend breaking down each role individually on a contract instead of placing all tasks under one blanket "General Manager" heading.

Staff Training: The Advanced Theory Course

If I'm counting my most expensive mistakes, staff hiring has to be near the top. Candidates who look great on paper, or perform well as athletes, don't always make great coaches.

In our glorification of the coach, we sometimes forget that "coach" isn't the highest-value role in a business. We can train others to be GREAT coaches; we can't train anyone to replace you as owner.

We also can't necessarily train anyone to be coach. After spending over $130,000 in three years on coaches who didn't pan out, I decided to stop looking for coaches, seek great people instead, and give them the chance they wanted.

The subtle approach has made a huge difference. Now, instead of signing people up to be interns, we ask who would like to learn more about the science behind our programming; about leading groups, and public speaking; about seeing what's on the other side of the clipboard. We don't mention a job, or certifications, or money at all.

At the end, of course, some interns will be offered work: groups, or their own specialty program, or some gym hours, depending on our evolving needs. But there's no disappointment on either side, and we get people for the right reasons.

First, select your best prospects.

Next, launch a learning program based on what you learned in the Level One seminar. Build in three phases: virtuosity, consistency, and intensity.

Phase I – Accumulation of Knowledge

Length: Four Weeks.

Classroom time:

• 2 hours/week (led by GM or Head Coach)

Training Time:

• 4 hours/week with other interns. No coach, just the group meeting to train together.

Assignments:

• Read "How To Win Friends and Influence People," by Dale

Carnegie.

- Choose a second book from a list of ten. Study and prepare to teach to other interns.

Phase II – Consistency

Length: Four Weeks.

Classroom time:

- 2 hours/week (led by a rotation of interns presenting material as chosen in Phase I.)

Training Time:

- 4 hours/week with other interns. Rotating coaching duties (Chris coaches Monday, Clay coaches Tuesday, etc.) The intern leading the group is recorded; video is uploaded to a private Facebook group for positive comments only (bright spots) to build confidence.

Assignments:

- Continuing study from list of ten sources. Add video from trusted online sources.

Phase III – Delivery

Length: Two Weeks

Classroom time:

- Shadowing in groups. Interns create appropriate warm-ups and demo while 'real' coach teaches skills and leads METCON.

Training time:

- 4 hours/week with other interns. Video review becomes more constructive/critical.

Assignments:

- Research of relevant material for in-class delivery.

Phase IV – Delivery

Length: Two Weeks

Classroom time:

- Role reversal from Phase III. Leading groups, with 'real' coach shadowing. Leads skill portions and METCON work.

Training time:

- 3 classes/week. Review is in-person after each class.

Assignments:

- Establish expertise in each class.
- Create content to introduce the coach as an expert.

Phase V – Continuing Education

Length: forever

Classroom time:

- 1 hour/month

Training time:

- As needed

Assignments:

- One piece of expertise-based content per month (written, video, lecture, Q+A, challenge, etc.)

When a coach is great, they have unlimited opportunity at Catalyst. Several have made a career here. But our goal is to create the chance, and give them the best possible shot at success. Their success builds our business, not the other way around.

Evaluation

Evaluation closes the "loop" of improvement. Rather than approaching evaluation like a sixth-grade report cart, we use it to measure areas of weakness and create opportunities for improvement. Consider it a Functional Movement Screen instead of a test result. It also helps to think about evaluation as the beginning of a process, instead of the end.

Using your list of Roles and Tasks, assign a scale to each Task (1 to 10.) Evaluate each task individually instead of measuring the "whole person." This will provide a clearer picture of a coach's value to your team.

Schedule regular reviews in advance (I prefer every three months.) If you don't set the date far in advance, you'll forget—until you're mad about something. That's not fair to anyone.

Start with a strong point, and then address a weakness (the most important part, because it's the greatest opportunity for improvement.) Then finish on another high note. Be objective and ask the staff member how they'd prefer to receive help.

For example:

"Becca, you're terrific at cleaning the showers. That's a 10 out of 10. I gave you a 6 out of 10 on your floor cleaning, so that's our greatest opportunity. How can I help make floor cleaning easier so our members can do burpees on a sparkling surface? You're also a 10 out of 10 on dusting; I'd like to get floor-cleaning to that same level."

The first evaluation with a coach might be uncomfortable, but you owe it to them to provide a running measurement of their performance. The most expensive mistake you can make is to let emotion replace logic with staff. Daily "pointers" will come across as nitpicking; saving up little grievances will result in an unclear, emotional outburst. And using unspecific evaluation will mean an argument instead of growth. People might not remember what you say, but they'll always remember how you make them feel. Regular, consistent evaluation is fairness.

How to Run a Staff Meeting

A box owner's exit from the corporate world usually means the shedding of both neckties and stuffy habits.

"No more meetings!" they say, and wander out into the great concrete-block unknown of business ownership.

Embracing the counterculture, they decry 'business-y' habits like a dress code; written policies; and staff meetings. As they're pulled into the various duties of managing, coaching, and putting out daily fires, though, a box owner begins to realize that running a business can be a lot like working for a business if they're not careful; if they're not leading, no one is.

In the long evolution of business, trends have come and gone. One that has endured is a regular check-in with staff.

An informal discussion between classes might be enough to share information or correct tiny details in a coach's habits, but it's not enough to set the behavioral tone, listen to concerns, or provide career direction. As a coach, you're guiding your clients; as an employer, your job is to guide the careers of your staff in the same way.

With a busy training schedule, solid staff procedures, and a profitable gym, it's easy to forget to hold regular staff meetings. I advocate scheduling a regular hour that's convenient for MOST trainers, and required for all, in advance. Commit to it. Don't hold a poll ("What works for you guys?") – you're not managing by committee. Set a time and make it mandatory. Record the meeting for everyone.

Like a class, it's important to keep your meeting to a tight schedule. It should start on time, and there should be clear leadership instead of meandering 'discussion.' If your meeting starts at 6, start talking at 6pm sharp; don't waste time stirring coffee and telling jokes. This shows disrespect for the staff's time

– you're wasting it, and if you're not paying for it, you clearly don't value their free time the way you should. They didn't leave home, or stay late, to hear gossip.

A sample template:

- Review of last month's goals (client retention, new clients in, revenues)
- One 'gym rule' on which to focus – usually your weakest link. Remind staff that the greatest sin is unequivocal application of gym rules, NOT the rule itself.
- "Teaching time" – done on a rotating basis. The staff member responsible for presenting new information, drawing links between existing pieces of information, and leading educational discussion does so.
- Choose a subject for next month's study, and a 'teacher' who will summarize and present what they've learned to the other coaches.
- Content assignments – give each coach one piece of content to prepare over the next month. This isn't hard: they can write a blog post about the subject they're studying; record themselves coaching a movement; or record a whiteboard talk about the subject, and you'll post it on your site.
  *A note about this: part-time staff members frequently ask how they're to be paid for this extra work. The smart business owner will draw lines between establishing

THEIR expertise and earning more money. If a trainer is renowned for his deadlift coaching, sharing knowledge on your site will create more demand for their services. They'll book more private-training clients, and their classes will be more popular. This works even better if they're not paid a flat rate for classes. I also realize that it's important to list 'content creation' on their job description, contract, and evaluation form.

- Review coaching points for one specific lift or movement. At this point, no more than 30 minutes into the meeting, the discussion moves from a private location to the gym floor. Coaches warm up and coach one another through a movement, comparing notes and cues.

- Staff WOD. After the top-down coordination of the meeting, it's critical for the owner to participate in the WOD to show comradeship. First or last, everyone should be on the floor together at the end. A small huddle afterword, for frank discussion of problematic areas, is okay; those go much better when the right hemisphere of the brain (responsible for empathy and group-relations) is triggered by METCON. I've believed for over a decade that most differences are best set aside when the bar is lifted. Barriers are broken down, and things you may not have heard otherwise are shared.

A monthly meeting keeps your staff moving forward, engaged and challenged.

It keeps your operation streamlined, and your group operating as a whole. It creates appreciation for the skill and expertise held by others, and acknowledgement for everyone's contribution.

The Big Problems (and How to Fix Them)

The Icon Problem

The first hurdle to replacing yourself in any role is to solve the "icon" problem. As the figurehead for your business, members expect to see you in every role. They view your staff only as substitutes of lesser value.

For example:

- Athletes ask which classes you'll be coaching, and book around those times
- Clients aren't willing do to some of their training sessions with another trainer
- "When will Chris be back?" is a common question in the gym
- "It's not the same when you're not here" is texted to you by a member.

These are flattering at first: you feel loved and irreplaceable. But don't fall into the trap. How will you ever take a week off without your business struggling? How can you ever sell your gym, or move on to a higher-value role, or make the time to improve your business?

If clients are disappointed when you're not around all the time, you're an icon. That's a problem.

"My clients think I'm their personal servant!"—Have you heard that one before? "They think I can just drop everything and listen to their little dramas!"—I've been there.
"They think I just drink coffee and surf the Internet when I'm not coaching!"—I've been there too.

When I finally realized that a stable income meant working ON my business, I struggled to separate myself from the day-to-day stuff. I wrote blog posts and read articles while sitting at the front desk of my gym; clients felt like I was ignoring them. When I expanded and put in a small office, they'd knock and ask why I was "hiding" in there. I was frustrated because I really liked these people, and didn't want them to think I was avoiding them…but needed to get things done or the gym would fail. I couldn't say those words because I had to create the impression of success for their sake. It took a long time to realize they were knocking on my door because they didn't know other coaches could answer their question.

The only replacement for an icon is a movement. Establish the expertise and authority of your coaches. Refer to yourself as one of "the team." Attend seminars led by your staff; attend your classes as an athlete. Take yourself off the pedestal.

A movement continues after its leader is gone. A movement feeds on itself, requiring little inspiration from the top. A movement creates its own momentum.

In a section called "Establishing Authority," I'll break this process down completely. For now, just be aware of the "icon problem" and start referring clients to other coaches for help. When you remove yourself from a role, hand it over completely, and let everyone know.

I had a booming personal training business in 2012: 30 clients spending a minimum of one hour each week with me. The revenue was a major part of our business. It was a risk to stop taking one-on-one clients, but I knew the only way I could devote the time necessary to creating a sustainable business was to cut back. I simply didn't have any other time.

It was scary to hand clients off to another trainer, but I started to identify some who might make the switch. I told them the change was absolutely necessary, and that I'd miss training them, but others were eager for the opportunity. Unfortunately, I forgot one detail:

"Why can you train HER but not ME?"
Because of my own "icon problem," I had to remove myself from personal training entirely. I couldn't pick and choose a smaller clientele, because someone's feelings would be hurt. I had to establish the expertise of my other coaches quickly, and then stop doing 1-on-1 training entirely.

You can avoid this problem by demonstrating the expertise of your replacements BEFORE you step back. If your coaches want a career in fitness, they can have it, and you can help by creating opportunities for "intrapreneurialism" and then backing away.

The Tuxedo Problem

Your customers think you're rich.
"You own a business? Wow. Can you lend me a hundred bucks?"
As all owners know, owning a business isn't a guaranteed road to anything but work. Most owners of small businesses don't dare calculate their earnings per hour, because they'd be tempted to

give up and work for their competitor. But most are BETTER than their competitor...so why aren't they earning more?

Sales is the answer. They're great at a craft--cutting hair, teaching fitness, giving advice--but they're not great at selling themselves, so no one knows about them. Their genius is invisible.

In late 2005, I opened my first business. Barely a month went by before my nephew--a high school senior--asked to borrow my tuxedo. I was bewildered: what tuxedo?

"Well, you own a business. You must have one."

At the time, I was in the high-adrenaline, don't-need-to-sleep phase. I wasn't making much, but I didn't care; I figured I could outwork anyone, and eventually my excellent service would be recognized. Clients would just...FIND me, somehow. My name would be whispered on street corners, and I would be sought. I was wrong, and stayed wrong for years.

When I finally admitted I needed help, I turned to the infinite library of business books online. I listened to audiobooks on my drive (almost two hours every day,) and heard thousands of hours of advice that boiled down to two words: sell more.

Simple. Except I didn't want to sell. Or more precisely, I didn't want to feel like a salesman. So I resisted, even though Zig Ziglar assured me that everyone--even Jesus--was a salesman. It just didn't feel right.

In "Born to Sell," Daniel Pink cites a study in which participants were asked to draw a picture of a "salesman." They all drew a caricature: the slicked-back, bell-bottoms-and-bad-sport-coat used car salesman. It's a sharp contrast to the image of a tuxedo-clad business owner, but they're the same person. They have to be.

Many owners are so afraid of the Used Car Salesman image they'll avoid selling themselves altogether. In fact, many businesspeople would rather FAIL than LOOK like a failure. They want the tuxedo, but don't want to feel as if they sold a few lemons to get there.

And that's fine.

Seth Godin taught me to tell stories about my clients, and that seemed better than testimonials. And Greg Glassman taught me to "be better period," but he was a master of showing off his expertise (more on that later.) These both had their influence, but it took me almost a decade to figure out how to NOT sell and still make a fantastic living.

That's right: you don't have to sell. You just have to help.

When children are asked to draw a picture of a "helper," they might doodle someone carrying grocery bags or changing a tire. But if you look closely, the helper in the picture is always smiling. They're happy to provide service when it's needed most. And here's the best part: when the chips are down, people are happy to pay for help. They're thankful the help is available, and it's almost a relief to trade money for a solution.

My first business was a gym. In the last decade, countless people have thanked me for helping them change their lives. Every one has paid me--sometimes tens of thousands of dollars. But in their eyes, they still received a bargain.

What's the difference between "helper" and "salesman"? It's value. If you receive more than the value of your money, I'm a helper. If you paid too much, I'm a salesman.

This book presumes you provide an excellent service. If you don't, fix that first. But if you provide value far beyond your pay; if clients thank you for your help; if your customers love you, but you're not buying groceries, pay attention to the second half of this book.

The Copycat Problem

In my city, we have plenty of knockoff "boxes." They're not hard to sell against: I press my expertise through content marketing, appear in guest seminars and use the other marketing strategies covered in "Help First."

But I'm occasionally frustrated when another gym owner copies what we do.

When we launched ConcussionPro, our goal was to help local athletes and coaches recognize concussion and minimize its effects. My partner in the program has professional athletes with long-term brain damage in his family, and we're both sensitive to the concussion issue.

So we started a "baseline testing" service: for $70, any athlete can be tested in a battery of cognitive and fitness skills. If they sustain a concussion (or even suspect one,) they can be retested for free. And then their recovery process is tracked until we know things are back to normal. It's brilliant in its simplicity (you can read more about it on the ConcussionPro.com site or at IgniteGym.com.)

A few weeks after we launched the program, it was copied by another gym...for $5 less per test. This wasn't a coincidence.

Worldwide, there was NO ONE else building "baseline" testing, interviewing brain surgeons and educating emergency room physicians. No one else was talking with coaches and players about concussions in our town. The odds of this particular innovation occurring twice in the same town are impossibly long. Luckily, we'd already claimed the ConcussionPro brand and made ourselves known to the experts in town. The "other" service simply pushes athletes to OUR service now, because they want the BEST for their brains.

But that's not why I stopped worrying about copycats.

Last year, another "business coaching" service for gyms linked to a blog post that was remarkably similar to one I'd written years before. I ran the text through an online plagiarism checker; the results were returned with a "Yellow" signal (meaning it was probably copied but minimally paraphrased to avoid a lawsuit.) If it were a college kid doing the copying, they might have been expelled. And I have a fantastic trademark attorney. But we didn't pursue it, because I don't worry about copycats.

In Spring 2014, a college kid DID try to pass himself off as me to other affiliate owners. An owner I'd never met tipped me off because he respected the free help we try to give gyms. How did he know it wasn't really our post? There were spelling mistakes. Knockoffs make mistakes that I don't allow myself to make. But that's not why I don't worry about copycats, either.

The reason I don't worry about copycats is this: by doing what I've already done, they're placing themselves behind me. They're making me the leader by putting themselves in second place. They're followers.

When a local "fitness center" began advertising CrossFit classes, I wasn't surprised.

My response was the usual one: an email advising against the use of the trademarked term, CrossFit; a phone call; and a rant to my Coaches.

We posted a plea, without naming names, on Facebook: "Educate your friends! These folks are NOT coaches. Their program is NOT the same. They don't care enough to know the difference…."
Twelve hours later, promises had been extracted, ads had been removed, and olive branches extended. It won't always be this simple.

As one commenter on our Facebook post wrote (and quickly removed): "Personal Trainers [at other gyms] are the 'sandwich artists' of the health industry."

Over a decade ago, Subway (owned by Doctor's Associates, Inc.) began renaming their fast-food staff "Sandwich Artists." The laughable title is still used, perhaps because the name is so uniquely silly that everyone knows its origin. It's branding by unintentional satire.

After all, calling a sandwich-builder at Subway an "artist" is analogous to calling a child's Paint-By-Numbers wall hanging a masterpiece. A BLT is 2 pieces from drawer #3; 2 pieces from drawer #5; three triangles from drawer #7; plus "Which vegetables you want on that?"

Big-Chain Fitness isn't blind.

They're well aware of the box program explosion, and will do their best to bleach it into their whitewashed system. 'Xfit,' 'Xtreme CrossTraining,' and 'CF Extreme' bootcamps are all on the rise, full of instructors who believe that box programs are 2 slices from drawer #3; 2 pieces from drawer #5….and maybe some pepper.

In our case, the offending "coach" legitimately believed that she WAS qualified to teach and offer classes after attending a "cross-training" course offered by a third-rate certifying body in Canada. She didn't KNOW there was a difference. To me, that's scarier than a phony coach stealing the trademark on purpose. .

What's our weapon? Expertise.

Sharing content – videos, journals, and articles – that YOU created YOURSELF. Establishing you as the expert. Sharing information – not flyers – at a high level. Hosting Q+A sessions, gaining the confidence of healthcare professionals. Knowing what we DON'T know, and working to fill that gap.

Competition from other Affiliates is not the challenge we face in the next 5 years. Saturation is. Start making yourself stand out, or risk being mistaken for "just another boot camp."

Fear of Failure

When you learned to walk, you fell down a lot.

But the first time you took two consecutive steps, your parents probably went nuts: it was a new trick in your portfolio. A big one.

A few weeks later, walking was a skill: you could do it consistently and on demand. You probably still fell down occasionally, but it no longer fazed you: it was just part of walking.

By eighteen months, you were walking up and down ramps, balancing on one foot, going backward. It was so ingrained, it was just something you did. No more thought required.

The progression from fluency to consistency to intensity isn't limited to fitness.

Learning to speak Spanish is the same: practice the basic nouns; put sentences together frequently; go to Spain. It's the same with muscle-ups, handstand walking, and your business.

Plan the work, and work the plan.

Planning the work with a mentor is a good first step.

But success over the long term means consistent application until execution is automatic.

For example, your first video teaching the squat is a trick. You have 30 outtakes, a choppy title sequence, and bad sound–but you did it: you have content. It's a big day. As you get better, the content improves and attention increases. Good for you: you're marketing. You can produce a video on muscle-up progressions on demand. Eventually, you get a GoPro and start shooting pistol progressions in Spain…

We're all looking for a 'trick.'

But the secret isn't one simple thing: it's consistency, then intensity. It's planning the work, and working the plan until it becomes automatic. Your first blog post won't be easy; the hundredth will be. Become skilled.

Owners of small businesses frequently don't allow themselves the freedom to fail. They confuse short-term failure with long-term failure; fear is an amplifier. They're terrified to make small changes.

Many of my mentoring clients will laugh when they read this, but a lot of my time is spent giving something other than advice: sometimes, I just give permission.

The typical "permission" call will look something like this, after pleasantries and metrics are exchanged:

Gym owner: "I have a big decision to make and I need your help."
Me: "Great. I'm taking notes."
Owner: "Well, I'm thinking about raising my rates. We have over 150 clients, but I'm not making enough to survive. Rather than dilute my coaching by adding 100 more clients, I'd rather just focus on doing the best job for the clients I have."
Me: "Great decision."
Owner: "The current members might not like it. But if I raise rates by just ten dollars per month, I'll have some breathing space. And if I make personal training an optional add-on, I think I can earn another five thousand every month. That will mean my wife can quit her job and take over the GM role at the gym."
Me: "Sounds great. What's the question?"
Owner: "Well…. should I do it?"

They already know the answer. I WANT them to know the answer (that's why I teach strategies instead of tactics: I want every client to know how to solve problems even when I'm not around.) They're just waiting for someone else to give them permission, because they're scared of failure.

Change is hard. It takes practice. And for many clients, I'm both the coach and enabler of change. Until they're confident in their business decisions, it's my job to help them practice. I can be a caddy until they're comfortable choosing their own club.

Now I want to give YOU permission to succeed; to take the risks necessary to be wealthy. I want you to start with small changes, and continually challenge your own confidence as your entrepreneurial skill grows.

My greatest skill is the ability to fail faster than anyone else. It's like a super power: I wake up, try something, learn from its failure, and try something else. I measure the result, and teach the "wins" to others. I do this several times every week. After spending 20 years making mistakes in the fitness industry, my failures are worth millions of dollars in saved revenue to other gym owners. It took many little "No's" to get to the big "yes's."

The False Start

Every week, we see posts from veteran affiliate owners whose clients are being "stolen" by new gyms, or being crowded out of their market by too much "competition." They're scared, because what they're selling is the same as everyone else on the street, and new clients can't tell the difference. They know they NEED to change, but they're terrified to do so.

The thing that made us special in 2008 is not the thing that makes us special now.

In fact, some gyms that were very successful in 2010 are now in decline. Back then, they were the only box in town. They were different; they were Seth Godin's "Purple Cow." They were remarkable. Now they're not; they're one of two, or six, or twenty, and no one cares that their gym was around first. New clients don't care. Passionate new coaches don't care. HQ cares, but will never protect anyone's territory because the pursuit of excellence means being willing to sacrifice what you currently have to make something even better.

For many of these gyms, the best first step is to figure out what made them successful in the first place. As they work through the process of peeling back layers, they might find many of those strategic advantages still exist.

Other strategic advantages might have gone away. That means change will be required. And it might be painful. But it doesn't mean they have to lose.

The vast majority of boxes sell the same membership plans: Unlimited, 3x, 2x, and a discount for paying in advance. But Greg Glassman didn't do it that way; it's just what everyone does because everyone else is doing it. Coach did it another way, and he had several folks doing Personal Training, too. Do you?

Many boxes don't believe they can add a Kids program, or change their schedule because...they've never tried. What if you released your current schedule as "Our Fall 2016 Schedule"? Does that imply that times might change in the future? Does it also give you the right to change BACK if you don't like the change?

Other boxes would like to add a better Open Gym program, but they've been giving away a few halfhearted hours every week for free. Why not start a better Open Gym program, offer it to new members as an option to purchase, and give it to your existing members for two months – for free? If they like the change, they'll buy it. If not, they don't have to pay for anything they don't want.

Finally, many old-timers (like me) have an inherent dislike of "boot camps" or other watered-down versions of box programs. The reality, though, is that we've hit the back of the inverted U-curve of attention: some people, after seeing the Games, are scared to try programs at a box because they don't think they can do it. Why not create a "step-up" option to get them in your box? If they're scared of the barbell, let them do it without the barbell at first. You can't teach them the truth if they're at the GloboGym down the street, and you can't change their mind in a single drop-in-and-try-it visit. Some gyms are even offering Zumba – the horror! – Because it's a very easy entry point for Grandma. She does Zumba, is invited to stick around to watch "the crazy people," and eventually tries programs at the box…

The pursuit of excellence is full of upheaval. Change is necessary for growth. Don't be afraid to keep your eyes open.

The Retirement Problem

Last month, in a room full of box owners, I broached the subject of retirement.

Few had given it much thought: it seems a long way off, and many are so focused on the problems of today that they can't think about the future.

In a meeting with my own mentor a few years ago, he asked me to list my fears. Though far down the list, the potential to retire (eventually) was one of them.

"Don't worry about that one," he said, drawing a line through it. "You're never going to retire. I know you."

What he meant was, I'll never be happy unless I'm busy. That's true. That doesn't mean I have to do the same thing until I'm 65 and burnt out, and then buy a big RV and spread athlete's foot from one public campground shower to another for the rest of my life.

Retirement, then, is the ability to stop showing up, and still be paid.

'Stop showing up' might mean taking a morning off to put your kids on the school bus, or a weekend to ski, or – in my case – pulling out almost entirely and doing something else.

What am I doing?

Writing, and loving it. Helping Affiliates through the mentorship program, and loving it. Putting my kids on the school bus. My gym (Catalyst) still pays me. I work about six hours per week there.

How can I do it?

I planned for it. I made myself redundant. I hired brilliant people, and gave them the same training I give to TwoBrain mentoring clients (after all, if I don't run my gym the way I tell you to run yours...) I promoted a coach to GM on Monday, and told her to fire me by Friday. She did. I'm 39 and semiretired.

I've done it. You can, too. There are no secrets to climbing Everest; you just need a humble Sherpa.

Growing Your Assets

The Cyclical Nature of Business

Education is the only solution to stress.

Lack of knowledge--the unknown--causes fear. Fear keeps you awake at night, makes you argue at the breakfast table, and gets out the vote. But some education reduces stress more than normal. For me, it was the autobiography of the Dalai Lama.

The story doesn't promote Buddhism, but does refer to the cyclic nature of things many times. And my experience, after 20 years in the fitness industry, bears this out.

In business this cycle is one of expansion and contraction. When preparation meets opportunity, a business can expand unchecked. But when times get tougher, the business shrinks down to its most stable point.

I've written several times about pruning a business the way farmers prune apple trees: cut away all that's not necessary for survival, and wait for sunny skies before branching out again. If the trunk is healthy, the tree can survive for hundreds of years. If the trunk is fragile, it will snap instead of bending.

As the business stabilizes with solid practices and procedures, the natural cycle of expansion and contraction generally shifts to one of momentum. First, as staff roles are formalized and mastered, the business can take two steps forward before meeting the next challenge and stepping back. As revenues solidify and become predictable, this cycle extends to several steps forward before one step back.

Awareness of these cycles can also optimize opportunities and minimize losses.

Five years ago, my cash flows were far more variable than they are today. I couldn't predict, from one month to the next, where money would come from. I clearly remember wiping my desk clean of bills in June, and considering expansion; then bottoming out my line of credit before September. "I never want to live through another August like that," I recall telling my wife.

Today, we can predict some cycles (like a slower August, followed by an explosive September) and optimize our own efforts to meet each opportunity. For example, where I used to prune back our costs in August and hustle hard to stay afloat, losing sleep and hair, I now know with certainty that September will see a quick boost in revenue. I take extra time off in August, and extend that same opportunity to coaches. When September arrives, we're refreshed and ready.

In previous years, when we didn't have a cushion, I'd cut staff costs in August and December; now we shift marketing strategies. Group attendance rises in September as families sort out their fall schedules, so we add coaches. We push PT harder in November, because PT clients don't go broke at Christmas. And we plan group intro programs in January to meet the rush; we plan Teachers' Week for the first week after school ends.

On a larger scale, market forces beyond my comprehension are always at work. I won't get metaphysical, but when revenues decline without an apparent reason, I don't lie awake all night; I just continue to work the marketing plan at the same pace, because I know they'll return to normal (or better) soon.

If you're down, you won't stay down. If you're WAY down, learn all you can while you're there, because you won't be back. If you're up, good: invest some as a buffer later. And if you're WAY up, solidify your base at this new level of net worth. Build another floor on your tower so when you fall, you'll still be above ground level.

Expanding An Asset

When I started Catalyst in 2005, I knew nothing about business. I was a lightweight who went into the ring swinging, and had a lot of lucky breaks. Ignorance gave me courage, though, and because I was unaware of the reefs, I navigated boldly.

When you're looking to improve your bench press, ask the 198lbs guy who presses 350. Don't ask the 300lbs guy who presses 350, because the smaller guy has worked harder to get there. He's tried more things; failed more often. Success has been hard-won, and that means more knowledge gained.

Many affiliates are finding quick success, and I'm excited for them I can remember, just a few years ago, when the discussion among Affiliate owners centered around the question, "What's your elevator pitch?" "How do we start conversations?" "How do we describe what we do?" "How do we even get on the radar?"

Well, the conversation is started, and some Affiliates open their doors to a waiting clientele. It wasn't always so easy. It will never be automatic, but enjoying 50 signups on Opening Day would have been a preposterous suggestion two years ago, and now we see it with TwoBrain clients.

The spot where most Affiliates become stuck seems to be around the 150-member mark. I won't suggest that they got those 150 by accident, of course. Knowing what brought them in, and what is keeping them, is the first step to attracting the next 150. Before you sign a new lease on a larger space, commit to a new equipment loan, and start hiring more staff, it's important to ask yourself, "WHY am I succeeding?"

This seems like common sense, but do you really KNOW? Are you succeeding because you were first in your market? Is your market huge? Are you succeeding because your retention rate is really high?

Doing client surveys, using a Case Manager and asking clients WHY they came to you and why they stay--that's important. When they tell you the answer, share it with others. This is another reason why telling your clients' stories are so important: their reasons for staying will sometimes be a happy surprise.

The next question: what am I earning per client (ARM)? What other opportunities could I provide without creating more risk for myself? If every client is paying $150 per month, and your gym is full, do you HAVE to expand? Can you create more revenue without taking on that new risk, hiring more staff...or do you have a $20,000 business that you'll have to duplicate four times to make a decent living?

Third, are your systems duplicable? Will you be doubling your workload by doubling your space? Do you have systems in place for recruiting and training staff, running classes, managing the facility and cleaning the bathrooms? Will you be fighting the same fires every day? Will you have to write twice as much, get up earlier, and stay later, or have you already filled those holes?

Can you lay your current business template over a new business? In more than one occasion, TwoBrain Mentoring clients have used the systems they've developed to aid another Affiliate. Sometimes, they charge for it – building these templates is hard work, after all, and this new expertise is valuable.

The success of new Affiliates today can be credited to the hard work of earlier Affiliates who struggled, attempted, failed, and tried again. If you're seeking advice, don't automatically assume that it will come from the biggest gym; seek out the survivors. After speaking to hundreds of these, I appreciate what they have contributed, and try to pass their wisdom forward whenever possible.

Growing To Multiple Assets

In the rush to grow at all costs, we sometimes forget to stabilize our base. A small gym with 150 members should produce a six-figure income for its owner IF it's built with the end in mind. Unfortunately, some owners choose to open a second location when their first is barely breaking even.

Here's my confession: I was one of those.

In 2008, we affiliated as CrossFit Catalyst, and I rented a second location. Our first was a Personal Training studio above a women's sweater shop. It had a high ARM because everyone paid by the hour--except the free little "CrossFit" group we were trying out in the evenings.

On the first day, the new location (CrossFit Catalyst) had zero members.

On the second day, we lucked into two: the father and brother of a Personal Training client.

A full year later, the Personal Training studio was still subsidizing the CrossFit gym. No one in Northern Ontario had heard of CrossFit. I had made the mistake of extension: believing everyone around me knew what I did and felt the same way about it. We discounted memberships and let clients run wild, doing their own workouts while a group class was going on, dropping empty bars, spraying chalk everywhere. It's taken almost a decade to correct some of those early mistakes.

Thankfully, our base was secure. While I made a thousand errors in the Industrial Park gym, our downtown studio kept us barely afloat. None of the errors were fatal (luckily) and the lessons learned were priceless. But the box almost killed both.

Finally, I moved everything to the industrial space. It was a calculated risk, but I had learned that consolidation often has to occur before expansion. This is the cycle of business: prune back the tree to its healthiest branches, and then allow them to grow without the dead weight. Repeat every few years.

Change is hard. Pivoting in shifting sand is harder than on turf, which is more difficult than on pavement. Without taking the sports analogy too far, the more solid the base, the easier it is to sprint.

As you increase your assets and grow your wealth, it's best to focus on one asset at a time. This sounds obvious until you have several balls in the air. If your goal is to own several gyms, the first should run completely autonomously before you open the second, which will have its own challenges. The second location will need your undivided attention: if you're racing across town between group classes or clients, both businesses will suffer. Trust the guy with multiple red-light violations on that score. Likewise, if your second asset will be a building, the first should still run without you for two reasons:

1 - if you get sick and can't be replaced, you're now jeopardizing two assets.

2 - you're going to need flexibility: in your cash flow, in your schedule, and in your patience.

I don't recommend large-scale staffing changes when you're buying a building or starting another gym. Some people can juggle two balls, but not on a windy day. Replace your GM before you start a second business.

When gym owners switch to a Stratified Model, there's some pruning required. Sometimes, clients don't understand why change is necessary (see: The Tuxedo Problem.) Pruning is sometimes painful (and also painfully necessary.) But without consolidation, the tree can't bear fruit. Fix or grow one asset at a time while the others maintain their course.

Three Points of Contact

A useful analogy for building wealth is the rock climber's strategy of maintaining three points of contact to mitigate risk.

When ascending a wall, a climber will set both feet and left hand solidly before reaching with his right. This allows for a bit of feeling, groping, and fumbling before shifting his weight from a stable position. If his right hand doesn't find a ledge, it's okay because the other three points hold his body in place. Three points are stable before one point takes a measured risk.

What are your points? If you own a business and a home for your family, make sure you have three solid points of contact before reaching for another:

Point 1: business. Can you predict the next quarter's revenues and expenses within a 5% margin of error?

Point 2: family. Is everyone happy at home? Point 3: house. Are you living within your means? Can you afford a short-term hit personally?

If those three are solid, go ahead and reach. Consider the next investment. But if any of the three are on shaky ground, firm them up first.

Growing Multiple Assets at Once

This is not to say assets can't grow without your attention. Let's consider four of my own:

1. Catalyst Fitness (CrossFit Catalyst)
2. IgniteGym
3. My building
4. My investments

While I work to build each in turn, the others sit on autopilot. Catalyst grows under the guidance of a rock-solid GM, who can lean on solid systems forged under fire. IgniteGym grows as word spreads, and Tyler is a very strong managing partner in that business. The building doesn't change, but its mortgage gets closer to ending every day. And my investments (primarily conservative, because no stock will rise faster than my own) compound without my interference.

If I were to launch another business, I would first ensure each of the above could survive without me: that they could pass the "Hit-

By-A-Bus" test. Plainly, if a bus hit me tomorrow, would each asset continue without missing a beat or wither and die?

Each could survive independently, and that's critical--but each also feeds from the others. This complementary business model allows growth in one area to boost the others. Unlike my gyms in 2008, each asset expands independently but stays in the same pie. In this way, the whole pie grows.

Consider, for comparison, an owner of three gyms. Heavily in debt, he's paying rent in three separate spaces and likely optimizing none. Without automation, he's running between gyms (killing his time) and probably not making an excellent income at any.

He's far from owning a building, or expanding to another asset because his first assets aren't really assets at all. He's simply bought himself three jobs.

It's common for owners of multiple gyms to make a decent income only through the combination of multiple income streams. In one case, the owner of three gyms--with 700 total members-- was just cresting $100,000 per year as net income, by his reports. Even with a 20% attrition rate, his gyms have to sign at least 140 new members every year just to stay where they are; that's not a level of stability I'd be comfortable with, especially with the necessary stable of 20-30 coaches, any of whom are likely to open their own gym within the next 12 months.

Instead, I prefer to focus on one gym with several highly paid staff members. Each shares the intrapreneurial spirit, and I create every opportunity I can to make THEM wealthy. That means teaching them, not directing them; and empowering them, not dictating. It means trust built on a foundation of understanding. Earlier, while talking about robustness, I mentioned building assets that feed each other. The success of one asset can improve or enhance another.

For example, if Catalyst improves its cash flows, it can pay the building mortgage off sooner and improve that investment. As IgniteGym grows, so does the pressure to "graduate" kids into our Varsity program. That necessitates more staff to help with transitions, and training programs to prepare parents and staff. Meanwhile, greater earnings can mean larger contributions to other investments, or the start of a new asset.

More than being robust, assets can become self-perpetuating if they overlap. Growth in one can feed another, and both grow at a compounding rate. I prefer to own assets that are complementary, but some owners would rather automate one asset and duplicate it over and over.

Duplicating An Asset

If your gym is fully automated, it can be duplicated. But not before.

Just as assets can compound on each other, time spent at one location will increase exponentially between two locations.

It's certainly possible to build a strong, self-sufficient gym, and then open a second location under the same brand. In this case, the brand is a larger asset than either individual location.

This means the first location must run completely autonomously, and should be tested. Can you, the owner, take a full month away without loss of clients or a decreased client experience? Will you lose income or net revenue by doing so?

I suggest this test for complete autonomy because of the compounding nature of time. If the gym's schedule requires the owner to coach five classes per week, that's only five hours of time. But five classes at one location and five at another isn't ten total hours: it's one hour plus a drive, then a return, and then another hour. Add fifteen minutes to each hour to meet clients who arrive early, and ten class hours between two locations can easily become fifteen total hours.

New gyms come with new challenges, too. Growing a new location from scratch will require time, even if systems are automated and coaches are ready to roll. Staff will have to be paid before cash flow stabilizes; can the first location handle the short-term losses?

"Stacking" services in one location minimizes these cash-flow and startup costs. Fixed costs drop significantly without a second lease; coaches can provide the new service during gaps in their schedule without driving anywhere. You won't have to buy new drywall, or meet new neighbors.

But if the right opportunity for duplication presents itself, a strong brand can be duplicated over and over. Though rent is often one of the larger expenses for a gym, other expenses—like coaching—can be expanded without being doubled. Here are a few suggestions for opening a second version of your first gym:

1. Have your processes completely dialed in. This will be the third time I've made the same point. Make sure.

2. Test #1. Go away for two weeks with zero communication.

3. Train more coaches before you need them. Don't draw your best coaches away from your first location. Addition of a second location shouldn't negatively impact your clients.

4. Rules, programming and payment options at the second location should be duplicates of the first location. Don't add costs unless completely necessary. Use the same software to manage both. Have a single phone number and one person answering for each gym.

5. Hire a GM, or take a managing partner for the second gym. Write a clear contract or shareholders' agreement. Reward them for increased net revenue. Don't make promises about "profit sharing" or "giving them a share." Put everything in writing.

6. Consider paying yourself as a consultant in the second location. Your experience in the first location is valuable; don't wait for the second location to become profitable to take a paycheck. Why put yourself on the waiting list over and over? If taking a partner, build your consultant's fees into the operating agreement.

Second locations can serve a purpose IF the foundation is rock-solid. Think of it this way: you're franchising the second location, not starting a brand-new business from scratch. All the hard (and expensive) lessons learned from your first location are more valuable than the location, equipment and shiny paint put together. In your first location, you're rewarded for taking a risk. In your second, you should be rewarded for taking the FIRST risk, not a second one.

Your Biggest Asset: Your Brain

If I've learned anything over the last decade-plus, it's to forgive myself. Yes, I make mistakes—often—and that's fine. Because I don't make the same mistake twice, and my mistakes can help others avoid the same costly errors.

You can learn anything, or overcome any mistake. You can outwork any competitor on an even playing field. If you give yourself permission to try new things, you'll eventually win.

My biggest advantage isn't my secret knowledge: it's that I can fail faster than anyone else. While my competitors slowly dabble with one idea over months, I've learned how to test a concept in weeks. I've learned the power of pushing an idea until it falls into a "yes" or "no" category; I don't spend time on "maybe." I can do this because I'm confident in my power to learn. I practice learning every day; I'm good at it.

Over the next thirty years, you'll have to change your viewpoint many times. You'll take punches. You'll be surprised, and often. You'll have to deal with ups and downs. My advice is to prepare your brain to think fast, fail fast and recover fast.

Your Second-Biggest Asset: Your Knowledge

Your world is now larger than its geography.

Your brick-and-mortar location is a delivery point: a place where you demonstrate and share your knowledge. But remove yourself from that gym, and consider who else can be helped by your knowledge.

Physical location serves a target market that shares one common need: location. They live near the gym; it's convenient to make your workouts a part of their day. But people have OTHER needs, and geography is less a limiter than it used to be.

If you have a particular area of expertise—a niche—you might have limited followers in your town. After all, there are only so many people who want to learn Olympic Weightlifting in Ramshackle, MO. But there are now eight billion people on earth, and most have broadband Internet connections.

Teaching is no longer limited to the physical classroom; a teacher's audience is no longer limited to those lucky enough to be born in the correct year. Your particular niche is probably shared and pursued by thousands of others.

Where once a unicycle-riding latex vampire was weird, we can now say, "There's a kink for that."

Kim Ki-Hoon, the English teacher in South Korea, made over $4 million in 2014 by recording his classroom lessons and selling them online. He's doing a bit of extra work—not much—but using his niche to help people. He's a better English teacher than most, and deserves to be paid for it.

I've worked with several of these Ki-Hoon-level superstars in the U.S., who dominate a particular niche but limit their exposure to a small corner of their town. Again, your horizon is limited only by your vision: if you're exceptional at something, who else can you help?

First, as with all service businesses, you can start by demonstrating your expertise. In the companion book to this one ("Help First,") the process of Establishing Authority takes up a full chapter. It all boils down to this: *no one else knows how good you are. Show them.*

A quick landing page with videos and blog posts is a good start. Talk about your passion for the subject, and share your advanced knowledge. Combine your experience with your education to provide a viewpoint that's unique to you.

Begin building your audience; track who's paying attention long before they're paying you money. Ask for their contact information in return for a special piece of content. Sell a book. Create "extended-play" videos with bonus content for subscribers. The hardest trick in helping others today is knowing who you're helping.

The Internet provides a great opportunity for a one-way conversation, and most websites do simply that: they broadcast. They don't build relationships. They act as virtual brochures, not the start of a conversation.

A landing page with a field for email entry is very helpful in this instance. By knowing who's watching, you can tailor your content to provide a more valuable resource. And then you can upgrade or summarize your service for those who deserve more.

After an audience is established, an offer can be made to provide greater service to those who want it. Some might choose to stick with the free service, and that's fine; I'm a strong believer in the value of free content to both the consumer and the producer. DontBuyAds.com and TwoBrainBusiness's blogs are great examples: there are over 600 written blogs, dozens of podcasts and a growing library of videos between the two, and they're all FREE. Businesses have been built upon the free cash flow calculators, manuals and forms.

Another example is TwoBrainCoaching.com, which serves fitness coaches. A mere decade ago, only the most experienced coaches dared venture into the business world. Their clientele was usually secure at the Globogym or University where they worked, and the risk of starting over was usually too great.

But today, ANYONE with a passion for fitness can leverage one of the most powerful brands in the world –CrossFit--for a tiny amount. For the first time, a coach's passion can outpace their expertise, and they can open a gym with a strong brand with minimal barriers to entry. It's a small-business miracle, and there are over 12,000 CrossFit gyms worldwide in 2015.

This means there are now thousands of coaches who know the fundamentals of fitness; who can take the average person and make them more fit than any professional could have in 2005. I was coaching for over a decade before CrossFit became popular, and I'll swear to this fact: a passionate CrossFit coach, even with a weekend education, will deliver a more fit client after a year than any University-educated "personal trainer." And these coaches want to know MORE: their passion for fitness exceeds the available literature in CrossFit circles alone. It's remarkable. CrossFit has saved weightlifting, will probably save gymnastics, and is taking over sport-specific training, too.

TwoBrainCoaching.com addresses that specific need. My passion has always been the science behind training, and TwoBrainCoaching.com will help deliver that science to new fitness professionals. Weekend seminars are fantastic, but can't deliver much theory. Instead, I can break up complex topics into bite-sized, five-minute videos, and help new professionals understand a little more each week.

I'm also leveraging another asset: the Head Coach in my gym is very knowledgeable (and better looking,) and can deliver HER knowledge to hundreds each week.

TwoBrainCoaching.com followed this general ramp-up:

1. Development of very valuable content to be shared for free.
2. An invitation to other professionals to participate in an online discussion around high-end topics. In our case, this was a Facebook group.

3. Shareable videos for gym owners who wanted help educating their staff. Also downloadable templates and documents.

4. A subscription service to solve a few major problems: gym owners who don't have time to provide ongoing staff education; staff members who can't attend meetings; and sole proprietors who don't have any other coaches to bounce ideas around with. This is a very inexpensive option.

5. A full-scale Coaches' Advanced Theory Course gyms can use to train their Interns or ATC students.

This isn't a plug for TwoBrainCoaching, but an example of helping a specific niche that wants more information. After coaching for 20 years, I have a viewpoint they can't find from their peers. And the platform will soon grow to include programming from OTHER experts, too.

Another example: IgniteGym. One of the first partners in Catalyst has a son with Autism, and we began a niche development in an effort to help. Over nearly a decade, IgniteGym has developed a worldwide following from teachers and coaches who want to work with special cognitive issues. We publish free content and host seminars (soon to be done entirely online.) We first built an audience with a site, then maintained the conversation through newsletters (now private Facebook pages.) We post daily

BrainWODs, and have since expanded into enrichment and tutoring programs—valuable additions to gyms.

The key to all of these is this: the value of the service FAR exceeds the price, and it's obvious. Removing the teaching of theory to new coaches saves gym owners valuable time. Adding the ability to help kids with autism will help gym owners perform a valuable public service (and add a large revenue stream.) But the greatest niche in my history has been mentoring.

I love talking business (and writing about business, obviously.) Since 2008, I've published almost a thousand blog posts on the fitness business, and spent thousands of hours on the phone with different gym owners helping them move toward wealth. I've done more talking one-on-one with fitness owners than anyone else in the industry by a huge margin (and almost a thousand FREE hours now, in which I even covered the cost of the call.)

This collective exposure, mixed with my personal education and experience, has allowed me to help hundreds of other gym owners. Some wind up continuing with individual mentoring; some choose the Two-Brain Business mentoring program. Each has a cost, but I've never been asked for a discounted rate, and EVERY client has seen a return on his or her investment far beyond the cost of the service. In some cases, clients have earned back the mentoring fees in a couple of weeks; ten times the fees in months; and will earn hundreds of thousands of dollars over the lifespan of their gym due to the coaching I provide.

In March 2015, I pulled two hundred of them into a private Facebook group. The new revenue generated by members of that group reached into the hundreds of thousands within the first few months.

This isn't an advertisement. You can do the same with your niche. Want to combine fitness with guitar lessons? Do it. Teach everyone else how to do it. Passionate about Obstacle Course Racing? Tell us how to do it, too. Enrich everyone with your knowledge. After you've done it successfully, we want to know how, too. Teach us, and know we're willing to pay to learn.

An Entrepreneur's Investment Strategy

In early 2008, I was listening to a radio show on my ride to work. It was before 5am (as usual,) and I can't recall the name of the show but have never forgotten the message.

The guest was a woman who helped entrepreneurs with retirement plans. Many business owners were watching the stock market closely in 2008 because they were worried about a trickle-down effect. Instead of portfolio diversification, though, the speaker advised owners to invest in themselves instead of the stock market.

"Think about it," she said. "Who cares about their business more than you care about yours? Whose business can YOU directly affect more than your own?"

A light bulb went off in my head--but unfortunately, it was just a quick flash. I didn't pull my retirement fund out of the stock market. I didn't use my savings to leverage an asset (like a building.) I didn't do anything. So I lost more than half my portfolio.

Ten thousand dollars invested in Catalyst in 2008 would be worth almost 25 times that amount today (calculated on the value of the company then against now.) With the amount I lost in the market, I could have made a down payment on the same building I now own, paid a mortgage instead of rent for the last eight years, and be pocketing another $4k per month today...and forever.

Every Sunday morning, I take an hour to work up to a "heavy single." I have a weightlifting platform and rig in my garage, and I listen to Jim Rohn while I work on cleans and jerks, and then snatches. Rohn is old school, and every 30-minute speech he makes provides one "heavy single" idea for me to chew on for the rest of my Sunday.

Rohn proposes a 70-10-10-10 split for your income. He teaches this split to entrepreneurs and kids, and if you don't have a better plan it's a great starting point. Here's how Rohn splits a dollar:

First, take 10c for charity or worthy causes.
Next, take 10c to invest in yourself.
Last, take 10c to invest in something that will work on your behalf.

I'll explain. The 10c to charity is self-explanatory. Whether you frequent a church and commit to tithing or just write a monthly check to a good cause, that 10c is well spent.

The second dime is to use on asset creation. Invest in your business, buy a building, start a new company or pay for new training. This investment should yield an increase in wealth: more money, less time.

The third dime is for investing in someone else's idea or company. Put this into a 401k, the stock market or shares in other companies. While I'm certainly not qualified to advise anyone else, I personally keep these type of investments on the conservative side, like index funds. Though I get better at entrepreneurialism every day, and have learned to mitigate risk, owning one business IS riskier than owning 500 businesses. Index funds are my "hedge": they're the average of hundreds of businesses.

Jim Rohn might seem a bit old-fashioned. But if you're looking for business advice, his audiobooks provide thought-provoking content. And if you don't have a system for allocating your income, his beats yours any day. Start with 70-10-10-10 and tweak as your wealth increases.

70-10-10-10 investment in time

Wealth has two sides: money and time. A wealth investment strategy would only be half complete without considering how an entrepreneur's time is invested.

In "Moving to Higher-Value Roles," I laid out a strategy for shifting toward a higher value for time. But there's a broader strategy that can be useful when starting. As in the money investment strategy, this is far better than having no strategy at all, and some entrepreneurs swear by this time ratio throughout their entire careers.

If you work a ten-hour day, spend 7 hours working IN your business. That means the actual delivery of your service.

Spend 1 hour working ON your business. Move toward the 10-Hour CEO goal. Start by formalizing every process in your business; then by duplicating yourself; and then by moving lower-value roles off your plate. Then firm up a retention strategy, and a staff education plan. Finally, master the marketing plan until it, too, can be shifted to someone else. Learn about ways to make your business more profitable. An hour doesn't seem like much for that huge pile of work. But hundreds of my own mentoring clients have started with 1 hour per week and gone on to totally transform their businesses into viable assets. Don't wait until conditions are perfect; don't wait until you can spend 40 hours being a CEO. That day won't come. Spend ONE hour every day as CEO, not coach or bookkeeper or Facebook reader.

Spend 1 hour working on YOU.

When you opened your gym, your job title changed from Coach to Entrepreneur. This is your career now. Doesn't it make sense to pursue an education in entrepreneurialism? Lessons you learn in your gym will apply to EVERY new business you can possibly own in your lifetime. Systems you build for this gym can be used in your thirtieth gym twenty years from now. This is why I sell education, not advice: I'm teaching entrepreneurs. Start with the books that appeal to you. Buy the audiobook format; listen on your way to the gym. My education started with a subscription to Audible.com in 2005, and has continued for one hour every day since. I learn while I drive to the gym; on days when I work from my home office, I learn while I lift in my garage. I enjoy learning specific business tactics, but LOVE learning about the mind. When you understand behavior--what drives us to action--and perception, marketing becomes easy. And when you start to understand what people WANT, it's easy to build services to help them. In fact, the first line of my book, "Help First" is, "What do people want?" There is a list of must-read books for every business owner, however. None of these were written specifically for the gym industry, and many of the ideas from these sources are translated into actionable steps in this book. Read them anyway: understanding the broader context will help you see the forest instead of the trees.

1. The E-Myth, by Michael Gerber.

2. Good to Great, by Jim Collins.

3. Made to Stick, by Chip and Dan Heath.

4. The Go-Giver, by Bob Burg and John David Mann.

5. Free, by Chris Anderson.

6. All Marketers Are Liars, by Seth Godin (actually, read everything by Seth Godin.)

7. The Long Tail, by Chris Anderson.

8. Second Chance, by Robert Kiyosaki.

9. How To Win Friends and Influence People, by Dale Carnegie (this could easily be at the top of this list.)

10. Drive: The Surprising Truth About What Motivates Us by Dan Pink.

I'm sure you can add more, but each of these will have an immediate and permanent impact on your mindset and your business.

Spend 1 Hour Doing Something Completely Unrelated.

Google's famous "20% Time" rule allows employees to work on their coworkers' projects every Friday. This is where Gmail came from, as well as other big Google ideas.

The "Two-Brain" concept means balancing creative work with logical work. Setting aside an hour each day to work solely on creative tasks allows for expansion of thought. This can mean working out; it can mean designing t-shirts; or it could mean designing a website for a new business that doesn't yet exist. During this unscheduled "recess" for your brain, you'll allow interhemispheric coordination to make connections between ideas. Many people find they have their best ideas in the shower or while driving, and this is no coincidence: low-level creative or "busy" work allows the brain to work through more technical problems in the background.

This isn't daydreaming: the ideal state of "flow" happens when the hands are busy but the brain isn't. Reading Facebook has the opposite effect.

Partnerships

I'll admit it: I've had both good and bad experiences with partnerships.

In a simple service business, where little time is required of its owners, partnerships are easy. When everyone LIKES the business, but none are truly passionate, there's no reason for debate; we just settle on an arrangement over coffee.

CrossFit Catalyst, about which I am VERY passionate, has always required more hands-on management. I have ideas often, and their implementation requires time and labor. I think this is true in the case of most Boxes, though it may not be so in other gyms. Both the load of work and volume are high and heavy. Heavy loads, long distances, not enough time…. sound familiar?

When a coach decides to open a Box, they might consider a partner to fill one of four needs:

- Money
- Business expertise
- Division of risk
- A push

In my own case, my early business partners filled all four. I needed capital; they had it. I needed business expertise; they were businessmen. I needed an excuse; they pushed me into proprietorship.

Occasionally, two or more partners might be equally passionate about CrossFit, and hesitant to shoulder the risk alone. While neither has an abundance of money, business knowledge, or overconfidence, they can lean on each other for mutual support.

"Partnership is like a marriage" is a cliché, but that doesn't mean it's not true. Like it or not, you're legally bound to these people (and perhaps financially dependent) so it makes sense to write a solid partnership agreement before the business gets started. A good partnership agreement saves friendships by allowing for a division, or exit, before things get rough.

They CAN get rough. For instance, it sometimes happens that one partner does the majority of the coaching, and one is responsible for the 'business side.' Since the 'business' work takes place largely behind the scenes, it's not always obvious to the coach. It's tough to value your partner when you're mopping the floor alone at 4am, isn't it? This is a small example, but a personal one. If we don't SEE them working, it's hard to measure their contribution.

If you're like me, and believe that consistency is important in a business, it's easy to fall into the trap of "I'll do it myself." When you pick up one task from the pile, you're likely to hold onto it forever, because 'no one will do it the way I do.' It goes without saying that this is a dangerous practice, and takes you further from your own training AND coaching.

Many of these pitfalls can be avoided in advance with a solid partnership agreement.

- First, agree how equity will be determined. If I contribute $20,000, and your contribution is time – coaching most of the classes, perhaps – what's our relationship? Are you my employee? Will we trade your time for equity – and how much? For how long? Will you have the option to buy me out later, or vice versa?
- Second, agree on roles to be performed. This means working through the business development process beforehand, as

we do in the Mentoring program. Break down tasks, group them into roles, and write my name beside some and yours beside others. Quantify the time to be spent at each.

- Third, choose a way to objectively measure how these roles are being carried out. Are you working enough hours? Am I creating enough coaching opportunities? Are you keeping clients happy? Am I keeping the bathrooms clean?

- Fourth, decide how we'll each be paid. I dislike the notion of an even "profit split," because it's very easy to spend money until there is NO profit, and thereby split nothing. If your partner prefers to buy 10 new bars this month to build classes, but you need grocery money, you're going to have discord.

- Finally, decide on the terms of a breakup. Before you look for a 'dislike' button on this section, hang on a bit. Chances are good that you're friends with your future partners. You're swearing to each other that, come what may, you'll still be friends even if the business doesn't work out. However, running a gym is a massive responsibility, and it can crush friendships. Your bad habits will be magnified, and my transgressions will cause you pain. Choosing a clean way of exiting your arrangement can SAVE your friendship. Recently, while drawing up the partnership agreement for a new company, my attorney recommended that we formalize a 'shotgun exit'. If my partner doesn't like the job I'm doing, or I don't like the job she's doing, one can make an offer for the other's shares. The offer is reciprocal: the other partner can buy out the first for the same amount. For instance, if I offer her $1 for her percentage, she can have mine for a buck, too.

What's most important?

In the short-term, getting your Box open. To that end, lean on your friends; make alliances. In the long-term, when you're standing on your own feet, and confident in the business systems you've developed, you may choose to go your own way. That's the natural course of maturation in business. Set yourself up to draw your own map later. After all, the vast majority of gyms ARE successful….and launched by people who have worked at OTHER gyms.

Investing In Others

On the other side of the coin, if you're primarily the investor in a business, decide in advance how your investment will be repaid, and how your risk will be rewarded.

The relationship between a "money guy" and new entrepreneur can best be described as "Investing partner" and "managing partner."

When I create an opportunity for a new business owner, I'm giving them a brand new life. I take that responsibility seriously.

Rather than "gifting" my investment, I believe it's the duty of the investor to warn the new partner of the risks. For example, if the business is losing money, all partners will contribute to the losses. If I own 75% of a business, and the new partner owns 25%, they'll be on the hook for 25% of the losses. Can they afford to cover? Will it put their family at risk? Would they actually be better as an employee with a sales incentive?

Likewise, it should be clear that their primary asset is their time. Cash investment gets the business to the starting line, but the race will be won on their shoulders. A business requiring a large time commitment isn't a good investment when wealth creation is the goal.

Charge a monthly "consultancy" fee. When a bank loans money, they don't wait for a business to be profitable before requiring repayment. Their risk is in the initial outlay, not the day-to-day cash flow of the business. If you're the banker, don't risk the money AND the time; charge a flat rate for your guidance each month. Or work out a loan repayment schedule in advance.

Finally, it's up to the investor to create repayment terms, contracts and dividend schedules in advance. A new business owner likely won't have the experience to do these things. While it's fair for the investor to be paid as a consultant instead of waiting for a dividend, it's fair to the new partner to show exactly where the money will go and when.

Handling the money, paying off expenses and deciding wage increases might seem like the natural domain of the investor. After all, the investor is the expert. But the managing partner is still a partner. They should help make decisions on money, or won't take the big decisions seriously. They should view the company as their own, with all the risks and rewards associated. This includes a clear path to buyout, even if neither partner intends to buy out the other. If the investing partner isn't happy with the management of his investment, he can repay the managing partner's time according to a valuation. If the managing partner is ready to take the reins, he should understand the path to buy out the investor.

Fairness means knowledge and transparency. A partnership is like a marriage: both people should know how to handle money and where it's going, or there will be fight over the food budget.

Growth: Good Debt vs. Bad Debt

Your grandpa is going to be angry with me, but I'm going to say this anyway: not all debt is bad.

In uncertain times, a strategy of consolidation is best: trim back non-necessities, and focus only on the reliable. But entrepreneurialism is, by nature, uncertain. We can mitigate risk to some degree, but the jump is what separates YOU from everyone else. It's that little leap.

We'll try to close the gap as much as possible, but that doesn't mean an avoidance of debt. Sometimes debt can accelerate your growth.

For example, let's consider the brick-and-mortar debt of a building loan. In this simple example, you buy a house and rent it to someone else. The mortgage payment is $500 per month, but you can get $550 in rent and the tenant will pay for utilities. How many of these houses should you buy?

Answer: probably all of them.

In the above example, the bank holds most of the risk, but more importantly, the debt makes the asset possible. If every buyer tried to save up the total price of their building in advance, we wouldn't have much of a real estate market.

In a more gym-specific example, let's consider the price of a new rig: if you don't have a rig, spending $12,000 on a rig is good debt, because you won't have a gym without one. The debt, paid out at $250 per month, should generate far more than its monthly cost.

Conversely, buying "the Worm" (some logs with ropes running through them, used in the 2014 CrossFit Games) probably won't create new revenue for the gym. It's not a necessity, and unless it will improve the fitness of your clients in a measurable way, it's a toy. If your gym has the cash flow (the profit margin) to support its purchase as a priority, great! If you're considering paying with a credit card, line of credit or loan...that's bad debt.

The key differentiator: good debt creates an immediate asset. Bad debt creates a risk.

Another example of good debt in the gym: a used wrestling mat costs $3000, and you don't have the cash available. But the mat will allow you to launch a kids' program, and maybe a Jiu-Jitsu tenant partnership. If you have a solid plan for a new revenue stream, or the asset will measurably improve cash flow in an existing revenue stream, it's good debt.

Now consider the case of a new owner who leases 10,000 square feet and spends $100,000 on equipment. He's hoping the "wow!" factor will impress clients to sign up in droves; instead of focusing on what THEY want, he tries to sell a ton of steaks (cooked rare.) Is this good debt, or bad?

If you buy a building to house your gym, you'll take on some debt. But your gym will pay the mortgage (and more, possibly.) Eventually, the gym will pay YOU rent instead of the bank. That's good debt.

Of course, even good debt has its risks. Your building could burn down! But we mitigate these risks where possible to stabilize the upside. For your building, you can buy insurance. For your rig, you can have solid operating procedures and a robust business model that creates opportunities for staff to make a beautiful living. When you have a rig, and space, your staff can begin the "stacking" process to create their own career. How can multiple staff members create intrapreneurial opportunities around "The Worm?"

Good debt can be leveraged far beyond its face value. Good debt creates an asset; bad debt creates only liability.

Conclusions

Turning Pro

I hope you don't need to read this. I wish no one did.

When do you turn pro? Is it when you get a supplement endorsement contract? Is it when you open a gym? Is it when you win a competition, or wear a sponsored shirt, or get hired on the L1 staff?

Turning pro is a conscious decision to no longer behave as an amateur.

You're a pro when you decide you are. This should happen before you ever coach a class: even if you don't feel like a 'pro' yet, you fake it until you make it. You model the behaviors you'd expect from your heroes in the field. You search for better cues, better habits, and better haircuts.

You're not tired. You're a pro. You're not hangover. You're a pro. You're not sleeping with your clients. You're a pro. You're not cutting your rate for anyone. You're a pro. You're not starting your class three minutes late. You're a pro. You're not berating clients. You're a pro. You partition. You're a pro. You're happy and excited. You're a pro.

When you fail to do these things, you're not a pro; you're still an amateur. If someone is paying you – even if they're paying

ATTENTION – they need a pro. Their hour with you must be the BEST hour of their day, or it won't fill ANY hour of the day.

Failure To Thrive

Profit isn't bad.

Charging for your time isn't "Nickeling and Diming" your clients.

If placed on the sickness-wellness-fitness continuum, most fitness professionals unashamedly guide their clients toward "wellness." They believe health equates to being "unsick." As gym owners, we know better.

So why do so many gym owners believe it's okay—or even noble—to run an unprofitable box? "I'm not in this to make money…" is the equivalent of your client saying, "I want to get strong, but not build muscle."

Helping people is your primary motivation. That is commendable. You can help more people when you're successful, because:

1. You'll be in a better mood.

2. So will your wife.

3. You'll be leading by example, modeling a healthy and fulfilling life.

4. You'll be able to train more and eat better.

5. You'll have the money to do more things for more people.

Personally, I've run a gym that barely broke even. Now it's very successful. The latter is better. More joy in the box, more novelty, and more fun. More careers for others.

You have the gorgeous opportunity to build a profitable business for a tiny commitment. A $3k affiliation fee is trivial compared to the licensing fees of a franchise, and many gyms see a gross return over 100x their annual investment. Better yet, the knowledge to get your gym to that level is out there in the business world (some of the best is summarized in Two-Brain Business.) Box owners simply need to put aside their self-martyrdom and pursue excellence in business.

If your business is breaking even, that's not success; it's volunteering. While noble, it's not sustainable. What happens to your family and your clients when you're simply too tired to keep working for free?

Dogma Vs. Data

In 2001, the outliers started paying attention to CrossFit. Workouts on .com were thought provoking. Coach Glassman was active in explaining his rationale with other sport scientists; his own clients and anyone interested enough to ask.

The earliest CrossFit Journal articles attacked the dogma rampant in the fitness industry. At the time, CrossFit presented the ONLY alternative to "body part splits" and "cardio." There were no bench presses or mirrors, and high-effort sprints instead of low-challenge treadmill walking. And now the industry is scrambling to catch up.

The real renaissance was a return to data: all the experts "knew" high-fat diets were dangerous, but the data didn't support the "fact." Everyone "knows" high-rep snatches are bad for the back, despite the growing pile of evidence to the contrary. Singular examples--Julie Foucher at Regionals in 2015--stick with us because they're dramatic, not because they tell the full story. It's just the way our brain works.

But the momentum of our movement has created its own internal dogma. Affiliate owners try to survive by selling group classes because "that's CrossFit." But that's NOT CrossFit. CrossFit means training people in the most empirically measurable and effective way. Data collection and analysis is critical. In a personal email from Greg Glassman:

"As a side note, it's funny how many opportunities arise peripheral to OUR cause of advancing the technology of improving human performance utilizing our uniquely qualitative tools (thanks, again, Sir Isaac Newton) for accurate and precise estimation of human performance. It's kind of a "duh!!" when you stop to think about it, yet a surprise to me. "

Some key ideas driven by dogma, not data:

"CrossFitters don't bench press."

"CrossFitters don't do biceps curls."

"Our workout is your warm-up."

"Killer workouts make for killer bodies."

"We need to include thrusters every week if you're going to get better at them."

"My retention rate is about 90%."

"We did this and my clients all loved it!" "People join CrossFit because of the community."

Where does data come from? Testing and retesting with the same tools. CrossFit gives us tools for testing and retesting: Fran, deadlift singles and 5k run times. After three months of training, a program will either make you better at one or two or all three, or it won't. If your deadlift goes up and your run time gets slower, the program is adjusted. But if none is ever retested, we specialize. We do the things we like instead of the things we should.

Coaches know this. But business owners guess. They set their prices based on other local gyms; they try a "free foundations class" and accept its mediocre results. Many don't know critical numbers, like total members, gross revenue, NET revenue or ARM (Average Revenue Per Member.) They believe tactics work because others--who also aren't measuring--claim they do.

"We made the change and our clients loved it."--How do you know? How many loved it? How many hated it? How much did they love it compared to something else? Were they presented with alternatives? In other words, what else have you tried?

Without the backdrop of context and experience--that is, without data--it's all just dogma. It's followership. This is not the CrossFit way.

When I introduce any new concept in this book or a blog or podcast, you can rest assured: there's data behind it. We've measured success first in my own gym, and then in a sample of others, and then in hundreds of the best gyms worldwide. While I give myself leeway to make a lot of mistakes, I don't take risks with other people's businesses.

You should feel free to take risks with your own, however. Consider every new initiative a "trial." Roll it out for three months, and give it your best shot so you're not second-guessing yourself later. Measure the results. Are you better? If not, try the next thing. Retest over time, because business (and fitness) evolves.

In another book ("Help First,") I introduce two measurement tools: Brand Action, which is a monthly marketing plan; and Onboarding, which measures the efficacy of that marketing. Both are great tools for tracking execution and success, but the real magic of data is that it reveals other opportunities.

For example, a professional looking at the Onboarding chart might notice some trends. While comparing a client's progress through the Four Stages of Onboarding, the gym owner might see clients choosing one-on-one training after reading the newsletter. Or it might be obvious that clients who use a Groupon don't stick around after their discounted "trial" period. Or perhaps a weakness is revealed: clients don't move from Stage One (Awareness) to Stage Two (Desire.) Whatever the data reveals, a gym owner can pivot their strategy to address opportunities. But without tracking, marketing is just firing pistols into the dark.

"You manage what you measure" is a business cliché. It doesn't sit well with entrepreneurs, because most of us didn't open a business to be a manager. However, on our path to CEO (and ultimately, "Perfect Day,") we must create systems and test them before handing them off to others.

Think about building a ladder while you're standing on it. You add a new rung; then you test it gingerly to make sure it can bear your weight. When you're sure it's safe, you stand on it to build the next rung. This is how our systems work: design, implementation, test, next. But many gym owners are still stuck on the first rung, because they can't be sure the next rung is fitted properly.

The mentor's role is to give you the dimensions and instructions for installing the rung. Then to apply a bit of pressure to make sure it holds up; and finally, to reveal the whole ladder. The mentor's job is NOT to show you pictures of fully built ladders, or drive a fire truck past your house, or talk about the ladder they're going to build soon. But that's what happens: shiny objects distract us from our work. When someone presents his or her new discount strategy or Golden Ticket Clearance Event, we're curious; we want to try it. So we leave the ladder to investigate. Sadly, many business owners will never stand on that first rung. They're too distracted by bright and shiny objects. They don't know that, from the roof, they can see everything.

Much of the problem comes from Fear of Failure. We're taught, mostly in school, that failure is "bad." But people who fail the most usually wind up successful. In my podcast, "Two-Brain Radio," I end every show with a "Confessional," which is a funny story about something I've screwed up. I'll never run out of material, because I give myself permission to fail. I try things, measure the result, and move forward with that data. And I try to learn from the data of others. Not the opinions, but definitely the experience.

School also teaches us that sharing answers is "cheating." So we keep data close to our chest. Unfortunately, there's no shortage of opinion online or from offline "experts" without data. Some repeat dogma; some repeat myth; some repeat me. All are wrong to do so without data to back up their position.

Over the last several years, and thousands of hours spent talking with affiliates, I've become better at predicting long-term success (yes, I'm tracking these predictions now.) Many factors beyond the control of the gym owner can influence success, so it's easier to predict which gyms will fail.

I can divide gym owners into two broad categories:

- Those who "should" succeed

- Those who probably won't.

The "should" category contains amazing people with the following traits:

- A 'growth mindset' (failure isn't permanent, education is most important)
- A 'game face'
- The ability work for delayed gratification
- A mature sense of "wealth" – they know the business has to be profitable
- A stable, supportive life at home
- "Beginner's mind"
- Humility

On the other hand, the gym owners who will likely eventually be working in another field share other common characteristics:

- "I'm not in this for money"
- "My clients don't want that"
- "We tried it and it didn't work"
- "It's HQ's fault / the other gym's fault / my partner's fault"
- "That other gym is stealing my clients"
- "I just need more people through the door."

Usually, even the owners who carry these ill-fated preconceptions can turn them around after a few phone calls, but some are fixed in their mindset. Those are the dangerous ones, and I wish them luck in their new careers. Box ownership, like group exercise, isn't for everyone.

Don't Quit.

In one week of July 2015, two gym owners in my Facebook stream posted that they were closing their gyms.

If you're in a similar spot, hear me out:

Don't do it.

The problems you're facing aren't unique. They ARE solvable. Others have been in your spot, and have broken through to create the lifestyle they want. I'm one, and I want to help.

I spend up to ten hours every week talking to affiliate owners for free. It's not a sales pitch; it's a different perspective, a sounding board, a glimpse of what hundreds of other box owners are doing. Yes, we have a paid mentoring program for those who want specific, one-on-one guidance. But my philosophy is always, "help first."

At first contact, most affiliates tell us they want one of two things:

- More time
- More money
- Both.

…And that's fine. The problems start with the belief that solving the b) problem will automatically solve the a) problem. It won't. You need a plan to achieve either, or both, or something else. When I started these programs, I believed that my 520 deadlift would automatically give me a big snatch; it didn't. One can help the other, but neither solves the other problem.

The next problem: the belief that the best way to increase b) is to add a hundred more clients. Many gyms don't have a solid retention system, and blame the new box down the road for 'stealing' their clients, or their former trainer for leaving to create a career for themselves.

Another problem: believing that staff members COST their business money, instead of MAKING their business money. The same could be said for time: if you can't train coaches to be as good as you are, say goodbye to your Friday nights for the rest of your life. And if you can't give them an opportunity to create a meaningful career, they're going to open their own box. But you already know that.

The last, biggest problem: functional fixation. "If I keep doing the same thing, nothing will ever change. But change means risking what I already have; maybe I should just do the same thing faster…" So you dig deeper, work longer, miss your kids more, make the same, and wonder why your clients don't sign a blood oath. Back to square one again!

Change is scary. Sometimes failure is easier.

Don't take the easy way out.

When an undergrad finishes their bachelor's degree, their commencement address always ends with: "…this is just the start of your education." It's almost a given.

But education isn't passive. It doesn't happen TO you. It's sought out, earned and then tempered through trial and error.

What you REALLY have right now is momentum. You're on the move now, if even in low gear. You're not waiting for ideas, advice or a "silver bullet."

My gym is called Catalyst, because my role is to be the added element that speeds up the reaction. As you now know, the hardest part of any movement is the start; an object in motion stays in motion until stopped by an opposing force. The ONLY thing that can stop you now is gravity. And momentum is a greater force than gravity. The application of the right catalyst can create enough momentum to land us on the moon.

Appendix 1: Affiliate Survey Responses

The 2015 Box Owners' Survey was the largest, most insightful poll of affiliate owners to date. We're proud of that, and you should be, too.

While some of the answers made us worry about specific boxes, we were pleasantly surprised by the overwhelming optimism shown by most. My first blog post on running a gym ("Don't be vanilla," in 2009) came when many box owners were ANTI-business. Today, competition has forced us to professionalize our gyms, and that's obvious in the responses to the 2015 survey. We're growing up. We're glad.

Proof: more than half of all boxes (54%) surveyed said they had a set of "written roles and responsibilities" in their gym. None did five years ago. 740 out of 917 (80.6%) have an Onramp or Fundamentals course; 88% of those said it was mandatory.

We still have a way to go, of course. With its low barrier to entry, CrossFit allows us to use its license without any mandatory business knowledge. That's good: we're now forced to learn these things to compete. For example, out of 1359 responses to the question, "What do you need most to create or enhance success?" 591 said, "More members" before anything else. In my experience (over 500 phone calls with affiliates, over 120 through the mentoring program, over 600 blog posts on how to improve, and a book with over 3000 copies sold,) this isn't true; most gyms should be focusing on earning more per member instead. But more owners realize this fact every day. We're getting there.

We'll address some other exciting (and crazy!) responses later in this post, but we care enough about the success of our gyms to give some tough love here. If you're not making a great living with your gym, look at yourself first. Other gyms aren't "poaching" your clients, unless they want to be poached; your coaches aren't "unmotivated" unless you're failing to motivate them. Your cancellations aren't all due to "schedule changes" and "moving away." And the CrossFit brand has a ridiculously high ROI: if you haven't generated 100x the cost of your annual affiliation fees in revenue this year, you're missing something in your business.

In the rest of this post, we'll review some of the biggest revelations from the 2015 Box Owners' Survey, and point you in the direction of help where it's needed. All the information required to solve your problems sits waiting on our blog; if you need more help, just set up a free call.

Question #1 was to measure the scope of our survey. Specifically, would the sample represent the size and age of the functional fitness business community accurately? Considering rates of affiliation over the last 8 years, we believe we're not far off – the largest group of responders, by far, had been open 2-5 years, followed by those open 0-1 year, and then the class of 2013. But our own market might skew those numbers a bit: at TwoBrain, we're frequently approached by people who want to start their business on the right foot (0-1 year) and those who have realized the business doesn't just run itself (2-5 years.) In my experience, the sophomores are most optimistic: they might have seen early success (and good for them,) or are hovering around break-even. Either way, they might still run the business on instinct for awhile longer. And that's fine.

But the veterans' responses to, "Did you feel adequately prepared to open your gym?" were revealing: in hindsight, 971 out of 1313 responders (73.9%) said they needed more guidance in fitness (13%,) business (31.5%,) marketing (25.3%) or something else (3.5%.) The "something else" write-in responses revealed primarily business-related needs (e.g. "Finding/hiring," "balancing life/work" and "a little bit of everything.")

The Bright Spots:

We knew we'd love the answers to, "Why did you open your box?" and we weren't disappointed. Most open their gym for emotional– not financial–reasons. 761 of 2615 (29%) responded: "I enjoy working with people and helping them reach their goals." Congratulations to all of us: we're in this for the right reasons. 408 answered, "I considered it a way to give something back to the community" — even more outstanding. These responses are what drive us at TwoBrain to produce hours and hours of free help every week. And that's why we push structure and business sense on you: we want you to KEEP helping your community for the rest of your life. And as a box owner myself, I know you can't do that if you're overworked, under-rested, stressed out or broke.

Most gyms now have some sort of "Onramp" program, as we mentioned above. That's great. But 338 out of 917 (36%) indicated that most clients start simply by showing up and trying a class. Only 225 of 917 (24.5%) spoke with a client about their goals before putting them into a group class. If you're charging a client to be their coach, you might consider a short conversation about their goals and history first. We say it often: CrossFit is for everyone, but group training isn't. "Free Trials" have a low close rate for exactly this reason: too little interaction. Unless they're already sure how your group will help them achieve their goals, you have to tell them. This might slow down the intake process. Maybe it should.

Pricing Onramp programs is a hot issue, and you can find advice on the TwoBrainBusiness blog.

WE LOVE that most gyms (721 of 904, or 79.7%) build coaches from within. It's a great start, and a more formal approach can only help. Continuing education will help even more.

Almost 90% of box owners said they'd do it all over again if they could. That was a huge relief: We love the business, love the brand, and want to see everyone succeed.

What Worries Us:

It's a fact: very few boxes will reach the 300-member mark, and that most will need to make a living from 150 members. That's reasonable and very possible...but not if you're charging $90 per month in a class-only model. And even those with 300 members aren't always making a great living.. Want more on this topic? Read, "Building a Robust Business".

Most gyms aren't offering Personal Training. 402 of 847 (47%) responded "0" to the question, "How many sessions of PT do you sell each week?" 284 owners (33.5%) said, "Less than 5" and 103 (12.1%) said "Less than 10." Of the 5 owners who said, "More than 40," I was one. Friends, one-on-one training IS the original model. It's the BEST model for many of your clients. And yes, some prefer it to group training.

Question #8 continues to be the largest misconception: that the best way to succeed is through recruitment of more members, NOT more revenue per member. In light of other questions, like 'How many fulltime staff do you have?' and "What's most important to you?" and "How many gyms are nearby?" this simply doesn't make sense. Read the comments, too: people know the best way to succeed is through more individual time with members, more time spent on business practices, and better development of coaching staff. Finally, considering answers to questions on retention, staff training and formal business practices, most gyms aren't ready for more members anyway. More members means more coaches (not part-timers,) more equipment, more space…since I've written about 50 posts on this topic already, I think I'll quote BJ Maucere instead: "…most boxes would expand if they continued to add members. I sort of think I will hopefully just use my 5000 sqft more efficiently. If I keep adding new rent, I never get to where I want to be. I'd rather cap my growth at 150 and then work to make more from each of those 150."

Almost 50% of respondents have a business partner. But only 229 of 917 (24.9%) had a notarized shareholders' agreement. Another 133 (14.5%) had a signed document that might hold up in court. 87 believed a verbal contract would suffice; they're wrong. A shareholder's agreement isn't a prenuptial agreement; it's the whole marriage.

The Head-Scratchers:

Question #7 had a mysterious answer, considering the response to "How many fulltime staff work at your box?"–a later question. While 450 out of 900 said no other fulltime staff worked at their gym, twice that number were sure they could take two full weeks away without consequence. That means many would have to depend on the schedules and priorities of part-time coaches if they ever wanted to take a vacation, or–heaven forbid–faced a serious injury or illness. Another point: some of the bills proposed to "license" fitness coaches in certain states would mandate that an injured or ill coach can't go to work…

Most owners reported spending "just enough" (58%) or "too much" (30%) time coaching, and too little time on everything else (branding-71.3%, marketing – 69.8%, business planning – 77.4%, personal life – 64.8%.) And out of 1954 responses to, "What's your greatest fear?" 1549 (78.8%) listed fears that won't solve themselves (ability to retire, pay for kids' education, bankruptcy, can't take a sick day.) Comments also strongly indicated a need for external help: ("Can't drive new members in," "Can't replace myself," "Being patient with member growth," "Chaos!")

Gym owners said their pricing model came from "What others are doing" 64% of the time (501 out of 778.) Some wrote, "What we feel is reasonable," or "Based on our opinion." In other words, they weren't really sure. And most also believed they were doing better than most gyms, curiously.

Finally, 48.8% said they were earning at least $25,000 less than they expected.

Clearly, affiliates need business help. But when asked the value of a business coach, about 1/3 answered "Less than the price of a new rower."

A gym owner in our mentoring program described business coaching as, "Indispensible…you should build it into your costs, like your affiliation fee." Another, this morning, said that his business had gone from 11k in gross sales every month to over 22k. And a third said that, of the 12 people he pitched his new PT service to last week, 12 signed up. All of them.

Let's be clear: these problems don't just go away on their own. Some respondents listed business-mentoring services (ours included) and that's good. We included those responses in our report. But the question shouldn't be, "Which business coach should I use?" but, "Which should I try NEXT?"

Any business service that will generate $1 more than its cost is worth it. Look for those with experience (they know what it's like to be in your shoes, and how to buy new ones) and success (they don't have to spam you, because they don't need the money.) Those who answered "no" to the final question ("If you had it to do all over again, would you?") were kind enough to provide reasons WHY they'd have stayed in their day jobs or remained a coach in another gym. The answer to every single challenge (not enough money/not enough time with family/not worth the ROI) is out there. You can (and should) make a fantastic living at this.

Made in the USA
San Bernardino, CA
22 May 2018